Priorities
in Biomedical Ethics

PRIORITIES
IN
BIOMEDICAL ETHICS

by
James F. Childress

The Westminster Press
Philadelphia

COPYRIGHT ©1981 THE WESTMINSTER PRESS

BOOK DESIGN BY ALICE DERR

First edition

PUBLISHED BY THE WESTMINSTER PRESS®
PHILADELPHIA, PENNSYLVANIA

PRINTED IN THE UNITED STATES OF AMERICA
9 8 7 6 5 4 3 2 1

Library of Congress Cataloging in Publication Data

Childress, James F
    Priorities in biomedical ethics.

    Includes bibliographical references and index.
    1. Medical ethics. I. Title. [DNLM: 1. Ethics, Medical. 2. Bioethics]
R724.C48   174'.2   81-3
ISBN 0-664-24368-1

For my parents
Roscoe and Zella Childress

CONTENTS

ACKNOWLEDGMENTS

As a rule, books are collaborative products, and this book is no exception. My debts of gratitude are great, and in the last note of each chapter, I acknowledge the specific contributions of individuals and institutions to that chapter. But some individuals and institutions contributed to the volume as a whole and deserve special mention at this point.

Many of the ideas in the following pages were tried out on colleagues at the Kennedy Institute of Ethics, where numerous discussions sharpened and strengthened the arguments. I owe special thanks to Tom Beauchamp, Tristram Engelhardt, Richard McCormick, and LeRoy Walters. Discussions with many physicians and health care professionals have enlarged my perspective. Drs. John Downey, Thomas Hunter, Jonas Robitscher, Mark Siegler, and Oscar Thorup have been particularly helpful. Participants in my seminars for medical and health care teachers and professionals, under the auspices of the National Endowment for the Humanities, offered numerous insights into biomedical ethics.

Mary Baker and Mary Ellen Timbol of the Kennedy Institute of Ethics typed earlier drafts of some of these chapters, and Wanda Proffitt, assisted by LaRea Frazier of the University of Virginia, typed several chapters in final form. I could not have asked for more gracious and efficient help from them or from two able research assistants, Dorle Vawter and James Tubbs. I am also grateful to Mr. Tubbs for preparing the Index.

Final preparation of the manuscript was facilitated by funds provided by the University of Virginia's Subcommittee on Research Grants.

This book is dedicated to my parents, Roscoe and Zella Childress, in gratitude for their unstinting love and support. My parents-in-law, Hadley and Pearl Harrell, have also been very generous and helpful. Georgia and our twin sons, Albert Franklin and James Frederic, provide my immediate community of support and remind me of my daily responsibilities and joys beyond writing books.

INTRODUCTION

Biomedical ethics has flourished for little more than a decade, marked roughly by the founding of the Hastings Center in 1969 and the Kennedy Institute of Ethics in 1971. Interest in this area persists because the moral problems are real and frequently urgent. While physicians and other health care professionals have to make difficult decisions daily, all of us stand to be patients or to make decisions about relatives who are patients. It has been suggested that we do not make very responsible patients because we have little experience with the "sick role." The success of preventive and clinical medicine has lessened our experience, particularly when we are young, with the sick role; and sickness, like death, has been relegated to remote institutions.[1] We might, however, become more responsible patients, and more responsible health care professionals, if we reflect more deeply about ethics in health care.

This book's subject is "Priorities in Biomedical Ethics," a title suggested to me by James Heaney. "Priority" (or "priorities") has many different meanings, most of which this title intentionally reflects. In general, it refers to precedence in time or in position. Specifically, it may indicate (1) a subject that requires attention before other subjects, or (2) superiority in position or rank, or (3) a preferential order (especially for allocating and distributing resources).

In regard to the first meaning, this book identifies five major subjects that deserve prior attention. Although these five areas of special concern in biomedical ethics do not cover the whole field, they are among the most important. Chapter 1 concentrates on a procedural question that pervades most health care: Who should decide? I try to answer this question by analyzing paternalism, a doctrine based on analogy with the parental role which says that professionals may legitimately override a patient's wishes, choices, and actions for that patient's own benefit. I examine what paternalism means, what is wrong with it, and when, if ever, it is justified.

While procedure and substance are often inseparable, the other four chapters concentrate on major areas of substantive ethical reflection: death and dying, research involving human subjects, allocation of resources, and technology assessment. What about areas not covered? Much of the area of genetics, genetic engineering, and so forth, can be analyzed in terms of the principles and rules that appear in the chapters on research involving human subjects, allocation of resources, and technology assessment. Another omission is abortion, which I have briefly examined elsewhere.[2]

The second meaning of "priority" is superiority in position or rank. In *Principles of Biomedical Ethics,* Tom L. Beauchamp and I presented several moral principles that should undergird decisions in medicine and health care: respect for persons (which we called the principle of autonomy), not harming others (nonmaleficence), benefiting others (beneficence), maximizing benefit to others (utility), and justice.[3] These basic moral principles generate other principles, such as truthfulness, and rules, such as obtaining informed consent from research subjects.

Even if we agree that basic principles take priority over others, we still have to ask which basic principles take priority when they come into conflict. One way to reduce moral dilemmas is to reduce the number and the strength of moral principles. Thus, some philosophers and theologians try to find one moral principle, such as love or utility, that can serve as the final arbiter, all other moral principles being reduced to mere maxims or rules of thumb. Such an option is closed to the pluralist, who believes, as I do, that several basic moral principles are irreducible to any single one. It is sometimes possible, however, to determine the meaning of principles more precisely and thus to eliminate an apparent conflict. For example, paternalism involves a conflict of the principles of benefiting persons and respecting them. But "weak" paternalism may be justified, because it benefits persons whose decision-making is severely defective or encumbered without violating their autonomy or insulting them.

Yet another possibility is that of establishing priority rules. Such rules would indicate which principles have the right of way in cases of conflict. They might take the form: Principle A has priority over Principle B under X, Y, and Z conditions. Such rules obviously reduce the role of intuition in the moral life.[4] But it is difficult to assign definite weights to the whole range of basic principles, at least in the abstract. One task in the following chapters that apply these principles to several problem areas is to indicate which priority rules, if any, seem defensible.

Sometimes we can determine what John Rawls calls a serial or lexical order of principles in a problem area. For example, in Chapter 2, I offer family members, physicians and other health care professionals, hospital committees, and courts as such an ordering of decision makers in terminating life-prolonging treatment for incompetent patients. Appeal from the first to the second in this order, and so on, should not be undertaken unless there is reason to believe that the prior decision maker is not acting in the patient's best interest. In Chapter 3, I offer a serial order of "intermediate principles" *(media axiomata)* that specify more fundamental principles for research involving human subjects.[5] Before the use of human subjects in research can be justified, it is necessary to determine whether several such intermediate principles have been met:

(1) There should be an important reason for the research; (2) there should be a reasonable prospect that the research will generate the knowledge that is sought; (3) the use of human subjects should be the last resort; (4) the research should have a favorable benefit-risk ratio; (5) it should have the subject's voluntary and informed consent to participate; (6) and, finally, the risks and benefits of research should be distributed in an equitable way. If the first four conditions are not satisfied, the consent of the potential subject should not be sought. But even if they are satisfied, the refusal of the subject to participate vetoes his use. Although the sixth standard sometimes excludes particular research projects, it mainly applies to the distribution of risks and benefits of research as a whole in the society.

My moral theory certainly assigns priority to the "right" over the "good." By this I mean that some principles of right conduct take priority over maximizing good consequences for patients, for others, and for society. Principles of right conduct constrain the pursuit of the good, whether that good is for one person or for many. They block our access to good consequences. But even though our moral terrain is not as barren as consequentialist and utilitarian pictures suggest, consequences of acts have an important place in morality in health care, as well as elsewhere. In the chapters that follow, I try to indicate how consequences and conduct, ends and means, relate in several problem areas.

The third meaning of "priority" is also important: a preferential order for the allocation and distribution of goods and burdens. For example, in Chapter 3, I discuss Hans Jonas' "principle of identification" for recruiting subjects for biomedical research. If we select subjects who can become partners and collaborators in research because they can identify with its goals, we have a priority rule: initial recruitment within the scientific community, then among the most highly motivated and educated and the least captive members of the community, and so on. In Chapter 4, to take another example, I try to determine the factors that establish priorities in the allocation of resources for and within health care. In particular, should health have priority over other goods, and prevention over crisis intervention? In addition to such broad questions of allocation, priorities also have to be determined for particular allocations: Which patients should have priority when a particular medical resource is scarce?

Chapter 1

PATERNALISM
AND THE PATIENT'S
RIGHT TO DECIDE

PROFESSIONAL PATERNALISM / PATIENT AUTONOMY

One of the most pervasive and perplexing moral dilemmas in health care results when the moral principles of benefiting the patient and of respecting the patient's autonomy come into conflict. Physicians and other health care professionals clearly have a duty to benefit their patients (and not merely to avoid harming them). This duty is derived from the roles they voluntarily assume and from the general social duty of beneficence. They also have a duty to respect the autonomy of the patient. These two duties involve both substantive matters (*What* should be done?) and procedural matters (*Who* should decide?). I shall emphasize the latter in this chapter. To highlight the important issues, I shall consider three questions: (1) What is paternalism? (2) What is wrong with paternalism? (3) When, if ever, can it be justified?

The conflict between paternalism and autonomy crops up in numerous cases, such as withholding the truth from cancer patients, the use of saccharin and Laetrile, suicide and suicide intervention, refusal of treatment, compliance with treatment, and involuntary commitment for psychiatric treatment. In all these instances, the determination of the physician, the health care professional, or the policy maker as to what is in a person's

best interest may be in conflict with that person's own self-
determination. Let us examine four examples in more detail.
Two involve paternalism; two involve respect for autonomy.

Case #1

A woman had a fatal reaction during urography (pro-
jecting X-rays to take a photograph of the urinary tract
after injecting a contrast medium). The radiologist had
not warned this patient of a possible fatal reaction to
urography, because this would have done no good. "I
could have told her," he said, "that there was a chance
she might have a reaction and even die. After calming
her down I would then have told her that she had seen
two urologists in the past week and both of them had told
her she needed urography. I have done six thousand to
eight thousand urograms in the past thirteen years and no
one has ever had a fatal reaction. We have been doing
urograms at this hospital for at least twenty-five years and
no one has ever had a fatal reaction. Because the indications for urography were great and the chances for a
reaction were remote I am sure I would have convinced
Mrs. E. . . . to have the procedures. She would have then
had the reaction and died and the fact that I warned her
would have done Mrs. E. . . . absolutely no good." The
radiologist proposed the following policy: "Our responsibility is to our patients and to do what is best for our
patients medically. Informing patients of risks and possible death from urography may not be in the best interest
of the patient and . . . it may be dangerous."[1]

Case #2

Janet P., a practicing Jehovah's Witness, had refused to
sign a consent for blood infusions before the delivery of
her daughter. Physicians determined that the newborn
infant needed transfusions to prevent retardation and,
possibly, death. When the parents refused permission, a
hearing was conducted at the Columbia Hospital for
Women to decide whether the newborn infant should be
given transfusions over the parents' objections. Superior
Court Judge Tim Murphy ordered a guardian appointed
to sign the necessary releases, and the baby was given the

transfusions. During the hearing, Janet P. began hemor-rhaging and attending physicians said she needed an emergency hysterectomy to stem the bleeding. Her hus-band, also a Jehovah's Witness, approved the hysterec-tomy but not infusions of blood. This time Judge Murphy declined to order transfusions for the mother, basing his decision on an earlier D.C. Court of Appeals Ruling. Janet P. bled to death a few hours later. Her baby sur-vived.[2]

Case #3

As a result of a chronic brain disorder Mrs. Catherine Lake had periods of confusion and mild loss of memory, alternating with times of mental alertness and rationality. Because she often wandered away from her home, she was involuntarily hospitalized in order to reduce the risk of harm to herself. Mrs. Lake indicated that she under-stood her condition and the risks involved in living out-side the hospital, but that she preferred to accept these risks rather than endure continued hospitalization. The District Court denied her petition for release on the grounds that she is "a danger to herself in that she has a tendency to wander about the streets, and is not compe-tent to care for herself."[3]

Case #4

Two sisters, sixty-eight and seventy years of age, and their husbands were searching for a schizophrenic daugh-ter who had disappeared after her discharge from a psy-chiatric hospital. While their car waited for a stoplight, a nearby construction machine hit a gasoline line. The spraying gas exploded, leveling a city block and igniting the car.

The sisters arrived in our burn center two hours later. The younger sister had 91 percent full-thickness, 92 per-cent total-body burn, with moderate smoke inhalation; the older had 94.5 percent full-thickness, 95.5 percent total-body burn, with severe smoke inhalation. The burn team agreed that survival was unprecedented in both cases. Both women were alert and interviewed sepa-rately.

The younger sister asked about death directly, looking intently into the physician's eyes. When he answered, she replied matter-of-factly; "Well, I never dreamed that life would end like this, but since we all have to go sometime, I'd like to go quietly and comfortably. I don't know what to do about my daughter . . ."

After she was made comfortable, the nurse obtained a description of the missing daughter and possible whereabouts. The social worker alerted the police to look for her, and telephoned relatives, informing them of the accident as gently as could be conveyed by telephone. The husbands were located at another burn unit. An attempt was made to arrange for a final conversation between spouses, but both husbands were intubated.

Meanwhile, the older sister doubted whether her injuries were as serious as reported. "I feel so good, wouldn't I be hurting horribly if I were going to die?" The effect of full-thickness burns on nerve endings was explained. The physician reiterated that he wished to do what she thought was best for her. She hedged. "What did my sister say? I'll go along with her decision." Since the patient seemed unsure of her decision, she was offered full therapy in the room with her sister. She refused the therapy adamantly but denied that she was dying.

The sisters' beds were placed next to each other so that they could see and touch each other easily. They discussed funeral arrangements and then, in the next breath, joked about the damage done to their hair. The hospital chaplain prayed with them. By active listening, he was able to convey to the older that her husband was not to blame for the accident as she had thought. "It's good to go out not cursing him after all our years together," she said. The younger sister died several hours later, after her sister lapsed into a coma; the older sister died the next day. The daughter was not located.[4]

WHAT IS PATERNALISM?

With these cases in mind, let us unpack the meanings of "paternalism" and "autonomy" and then determine how we might resolve cases in which they come into conflict. Both terms are drawn from other areas in order to describe health care. "Autonomy" is drawn from politics, where it refers to the independent self-rule of states without external interference. Obviously, it can be applied to many different roles and activities. For example, we could talk about professional autonomy, and, indeed, one mark of a profession is some degree of autonomy. "Paternalism" is drawn from the role of the father in the family, and even though it might be desirable to replace it with a nonsexist term such as "parentalism," the usage is so well established that I shall continue it. Paternalism, according to the *Oxford English Dictionary,* is "the principle and practice of paternal administration; government as by a father; the claim or attempt to supply the needs or to regulate the life of a nation or community in the same way as a father does those of his children."

What does this paternal, or parental, analogy suggest about the role of the physician or other health care professional? First, the parent's motivation and intentions are assumed to be benevolent, to be aimed at the child's welfare. Secondly, the parent makes all or at least some of the decisions regarding that welfare. When this analogy is applied to health care, the professional is thus viewed as benevolent but also as treating the patient as a child who cannot be permitted to determine his or her own welfare or the means to it. What makes paternalism morally interesting is the conflict of moral principles manifest in the paternalist's claims to act on a person's behalf but not at that person's behest. Indeed, the "beneficiary" of the paternalist's actions may even oppose them. The "beneficiary's" autonomy conflicts with the paternalist's conception of his or her welfare. The paternalist refuses to acquiesce in a person's wishes, choices, and actions for that person's own good.

Naturally, many health care professionals are uncomfortable with paternalistic authority. But paternalism often is the best clue to the framework of ideas behind many policies and practices in health care. Sociologist Talcott Parsons' classic description of the "sick role" illustrates the point. Parsons argues that

being sick is not merely a condition of the organism or personality but also a set of institutionalized expectations involving
several rights and responsibilities. The sick person is regarded
as a victim and hence not at fault. He or she is exempted from
ordinary daily responsibilities and is expected to seek help
from health care personnel. The patient's entry into the health
care system is an implicit acknowledgment that health is a good
and sickness an evil and that "measures should be taken to
maximize the chances to facilitate recovery or, if the condition
is chronic . . . , to subject it to proper 'management.' "

By contrast, the role of the health care professional is
marked by the presumption of competence, ability, and skills.
The health care professional is "a genuine *trustee* of the health
interests" of patients. He or she is also assumed to have *"moral
authority,* grounded in the common assumption of health care
agents and sick people that health is a good thing and illness
by and large a bad thing, and that the balance should, insofar
as it is feasible, be altered in the direction of maximizing the
levels of health and minimizing the incidence of illness." Since
illness is viewed as deviance, the role of the health care professional even involves "social control." Although Parsons
stresses that the sick role includes active participation, at least
to the extent of seeking and cooperating in treatment, it is still
mainly passive. For Parsons, there is no way to eliminate the
irreducible "element of inequality" in the relationship between professional and patient. This inequality permits Parsons to draw on the analogies with parent-child and teacher-
pupil relationships.[5] Finally, father knows best!

Parsons' model assumes that there is a shared value of health
and disvalue of disease or illness. While this is, no doubt, true
in general terms, there may be serious disagreement about the
meaning of health and disease; for example, masturbation was
once considered a disease. This model also overlooks the *value*
of health relative to other values such as eternal salvation or
the preservation of a certain life-style. Although the putatively
shared value of health and the physician's competence, skills,

and ability give substance to the role of "moral authority," this can be challenged in the light of the variety of definitions and valuations of health. Since the patient's own health and value systems are at stake, he or she should have "moral authority" superior to the physician's. Otherwise, the patient is truly treated as a child, and his or her dignity is not respected.

WHAT IS WRONG WITH PATERNALISM?

But is there anything really wrong with paternalism? After all, the paternalist is benevolent, and refuses to acquiesce in a patient's wishes, choices, and actions for that patient's best interest. Paternalism clearly rests on the principle of love for the neighbor in our religious traditions and on the duty to benefit the patient in the Hippocratic tradition of medicine. But I would argue it is still wrong, other things being equal. One argument for my position is the absence of shared values. Another involves the controversial claim that individuals know their own interests better than anyone else. Yet another argument appeals to the dangers of abuse if we legitimate paternalism. Although these arguments should not be dismissed, there is another that is even more persuasive: individuals have certain rights in regard to both what should be done and who should decide, and paternalist health care usually violates them. The patient's *needs,* as defined by the professional, cannot cancel the patient's substantive and procedural *rights.*

To see why paternalism is prima facie wrong, we need to distinguish it as clearly as possible from other reasons for refusing to acquiesce in a person's wishes, choices, and actions. We might, for example, override one person's autonomy in order (*a*) to prevent harm to another person, (*b*) to prevent the person from imposing unfair burdens on others, or (*c*) to prevent the violation of other moral principles. All these reasons for overriding a person's liberty appeal to some object other than that person's own interests, or welfare, and thus they are not paternalistic. Obviously, many decisions in health care and public policy involve a mixture of these and other reasons, as in the debates over requiring motorcyclists to wear helmets.

Liberty is what Robert Nozick calls a "side-constraint" on our actions toward others.[6] It constrains our pursuit of valuable goals for ourselves, for others, and even for the one whose liberty is at stake. But exactly what this side-constraint means will not be clear unless we distinguish two conceptions of liberty. Liberty is sometimes viewed as *license,* as the freedom to do whatever one wants to do. All interferences, including paternalistic interferences, would be at least prima facie wrong, but they could be justified under some circumstances —for example, when others are injured. Ronald Dworkin suggests that liberty as license may be too broad because it encompasses acts we think people have no right to perform and implies that every interference with a person's wishes, choices, and actions involves a conflict between liberty and some other value. Dworkin argues that there is no right to liberty if we interpret liberty as license. Furthermore, the appeal to liberty as license is too easy, because it allows us to avoid determining exactly what is wrong with paternalistic interventions.

If liberty as license is inadequate, what Dworkin calls liberty as *independence* is more satisfactory. This conception of liberty focuses on "the status of a person as independent and equal rather than subservient." Liberty as license is an indiscriminate concept in that it does not distinguish among liberties. Liberty is liberty, and each liberty is on the same level as any other. Liberty as independence, however, distinguishes among and ranks various liberties according to their importance. Such a ranking would depend on the general requirement of equal concern and respect. As Dworkin interprets John Stuart Mill, "laws that constrain one man, on the sole ground that he is incompetent to decide what is right for himself, are profoundly insulting to him. They make him intellectually and morally subservient to the conformists who form the majority, and deny him the independence to which he is entitled."[7] Thus, the important moral concepts for many political and other matters are personality, dignity, and insult.

Much of this analysis properly applies to the sphere of health care, especially to relationships between health care professionals and patients. These narrower relationships, like their more general counterparts, involve power and control: Who may do what to whom? We have little difficulty, I think, in determining that a person's liberty (as license) in health care matters may be curtailed in order to prevent harm to others. Similarly, liberty (as independence) does not include the right to harm others and thus is not violated by some restrictions on choices and actions. (See Case #2, in which the transfusion was ordered for the infant.) Thus, regardless of which view of liberty we hold, we arrive at the same point: restrictions under some conditions are justified.

Either approach can provide a strong argument against paternalism. The ground offered by liberty as license is clear enough: any curtailment of liberty, any interference with wishes, choices, and actions, requires justification. To prevent harm or injustice to others or to the society is sufficient justification. What ground is offered by liberty as independence? When a refusal to accept a person's wishes, choices, and actions is based on protecting others, that person is not *insulted* or treated with *indignity.* That person is insulted, however, when his or her wishes, choices, or actions are simply ignored or overridden. In short, a professional's refusal to acquiesce in a patient's wishes, choices, and actions, *where no one else is involved,* and merely because the professional disagrees with the patient's values, is a profound affront to dignity and independence. It makes one person subservient to another person's conception of the good. The patient loses his or her independence and status as an equal. Paternalism is insulting because it treats the patient as a child, i.e., as one who has not yet formed a conception of good and evil, of benefits and harms, or is not able to act on that conception in these circumstances. Paternalism is morally suspect because of its *reason* for interference with a person's wishes, choices, and actions. There is a value attached to a person's freedom to make important choices (such as consent to or refusal of medical treatment) and to a person's right to make such choices. Social recognition of an individual's entitlement to make certain choices is a symbolic expression of respect for persons.

WHEN IS PATERNALISM JUSTIFIED?

My argument up to this point does not establish that paternalism is never justified, but only that it is prima facie wrong and thus needs to be justified. It can be justified under some conditions. For example, paternalistic interventions with regard to children are often justified because children are incompetent in certain areas and are exposed to risk of harm. This example provides two sorts of justification often given for paternalistic interventions: (1) the patient's defects, encumbrances, and limitations, and (2) the probability and amount of harm. If the first of these conditions is held to be necessary for justified paternalism, the position is "weak" paternalism. Weak paternalism allows intervention only where wishes, choices, or actions are not fully voluntary because of incompetence, ignorance, or some internal or external constraint. If, however, the second set of conditions—the probability of harm—is sufficient to justify paternalism, the position is "strong" paternalism.[8] According to strong paternalism, intervention can be justified when a patient's analysis of risks and benefits is unreasonable even though his or her wishes, choices, or actions are informed and voluntary.

I am inclined to consider these two conditions as jointly necessary for justified paternalism. Let us assume a situation in which no one other than the patient is at risk. If there is incompetence, lack of information, or involuntariness on the part of the patient, we can still justify intervention *only* when it is necessary to prevent harm to the one whose freedom is restricted. A person may be incompetent in one area but not in others. Professionals and the society should not intervene in all the person's affairs unless it is necessary to do so in order to prevent harm. Where only the patient is at risk, with no sign of incompetence, ignorance, or involuntariness, generally we should not intervene. In Case #2, the judge determined that Janet P., a practicing Jehovah's Witness, was indeed competent to refuse transfusions, and that her action was not irrational in relation to her beliefs regarding salvation and continued existence. Even though she subjected herself to the risk of death, and subsequently died, accepting the risk of death was not, by itself, a sufficient reason to override her choice.

While these two conditions are jointly necessary for justified paternalism, they are not sufficient. Although I shall concentrate on these two conditions, others need to be identified. It is not enough to show that there is a risk of serious harm to a person who is, for example, incompetent. The paternalistic decision maker should also show that the harm to be prevented or the benefit to be provided really outweighs the loss of independence and any other benefits the patient seeks in taking the risks in question. Paternalistic intervention should have a reasonable chance to prevent the harm, and it should be the last resort, employed only after other measures have proved ineffective. Finally, the least restrictive and insulting means should be employed. Among the various ways to reduce risk-taking, such as providing information, giving advice, offering incentives, manipulating, and coercing, some clearly pose less serious moral issues than others.

I can address the four cases here only in terms of the first two conditions, with occasional reference to some of the others. In Case #1, the radiologist unjustifiably withheld information regarding the possibility of a fatal reaction to urography. His patient apparently did not suffer from any limitations that would have justified withholding information, and the risk (e.g., from anxiety) was not sufficient to warrant nondisclosure.

In Case #2, the judge rightly allowed Janet P. to exercise her autonomy by assuming the risk of death through refusing a blood transfusion even while rightly authorizing transfusions for her infant. As long as she suffered from no defect or limitation on her capacity to make decisions, her choice to assume the risk of death in order to achieve salvation should not be overridden. Nevertheless, Jehovah's Witness cases can be complicated. Some patients refuse to *consent* to transfusions but appear not to view court-ordered transfusions as their own responsibility. In a Georgetown Hospital case, the judge found a way both to protect the woman's conscience and to save her life. Having determined that she could not consent to a transfusion and yet did not want to die, he ordered a transfusion for which she would not see herself responsible.[9]

This last case suggests the inadequacy of another condition that some have held is necessary for justified paternalism. John Rawls, for instance, holds that to justify paternalism "we must be able to argue that with the development or the recovery of his rational powers the individual in question will accept our decision on his behalf and agree with us that we did the best thing for him."[10] For this view—which I call a "ratification theory" since the patient ratifies the action on his or her behalf —the patient's future consent is a necessary (though not a sufficient) condition for justified paternalism. But in the Georgetown Hospital case, the patient's future consent was precluded by her religious beliefs. The strategy used in this case will not work, however, for those Jehovah's Witnesses whose consciences impose strict liabilities so that what is prohibited is not only consent but also the transfusion itself. They hold that the transfusion contaminates the patient regardless of consent or refusal.

In Case #3, there were debates about both Mrs. Lake's competence and her risk of harm. From the available evidence it appears that her freedom was unjustifiably restricted.

Even if the standards I have identified are acceptable, they do not always provide clear answers. This point is illustrated by the continuing controversy over the treatment of severely burned patients. Case #4 was drawn from an article, "Autonomy for Burned Patients When Survival Is Unprecedented," in *The New England Journal of Medicine*. [11] The authors, members of the burn team for L.A. County-USC Medical Center, hold that "during the first few hours of hospitalization . . . even the most severely burned patient is usually alert and mentally competent." Thus, the burn team takes what the authors describe as "an *aggressive* approach to decision making to preserve patient autonomy" (my italics). Patients are given sufficient information about their condition and prospects and are asked whether they wish to choose between full therapy and ordinary care. The authors contend that such patients both exercise more "self-determination" and receive more "empathy" and that their mortality rates have not increased.

Needless to say, this "aggressive approach" toward autonomy is controversial. First, it does not merely respect autonomy; it actively promotes autonomy under most difficult conditions. Second, critics of the report have argued that the burn victim is under "physical and emotional shock" even in the early period and thus cannot really participate in decision-making.[12] These critics hold that the first condition for justified paternalism is met in these cases. Third, some also hold that "there have been instances in which patients with as much as 90%–95% third degree burns have been salvaged."[13] But withholding therapy at the patient's request guarantees death. In short, controversy rages about both of the first two conditions for justified paternalism: limitations on the patient's capacity to make decisions and the risks of harm to the patient.

Finally, cases like these often involve a serious problem of communication. In the well-known Texas burn case, a very athletic young man was severely burned; after several months of therapy and various operations, he asked to be allowed to die.[14] In videotaped conversations, this young man appears to be competent, rational, lucid, and determined to die, with good reasons, given his goals and prospects. However, once his right to die was finally acknowledged, he chose not to exercise it. Perhaps his earlier demand to be allowed to die was mainly a protest against fate, against a loss of control over his destiny, or against what he construed as depersonalized care. He did not really mean that he wanted to die, but he wanted the right to make that decision for himself.

PROCEDURES AND SYMBOLS

Let me now indicate the importance of procedures and of the symbolic expression of values in relation not only to specific actions but also to medical practices. I have argued here that paternalism is prima facie wrong but that some instances of weak paternalism can be morally justified. The moral presumption against paternalism derives from our duty to respect persons as equals and the correlative right of persons to be treated as equals. While this moral presumption is built into some medical practices, such as the eliciting of informed consent at certain stages in treatment and research, many medical practices presume paternalism except where questions are raised. As Wendy Carlton, a sociologist, emphasizes,

> Unless one of the parties to a clinical decision makes explicit the lack of value consensus, as when the patient asserts religious beliefs, the illusion of consensus will be assumed and maintained. In particular, the physician's judgment of what is in the best interest of the patient will be offered and accepted, unless the patient or the hospital administrator [or some other agent] is prepared to challenge the physician.[15]

It is important, then, to cultivate an ethos and to establish practices with clear presumptions in favor of patient autonomy.[16] In particular, it is important to establish procedures of moral reasoning and moral accountability. These would affirm the priority of patient autonomy but would also indicate the conditions under which a patient's wishes, choices, and actions could be overridden.

The procedures of moral reasoning, which should be inculcated in the medical ethos and specified in institutional standards, should involve exactly the sorts of conditions I specified earlier when I considered the selective justification of paternalism. The procedures of accountability should specify both institutional agents and mechanisms for determining when the conditions are present for justifiably overriding the patient's wishes, choices, and actions. Responsibility could be diffused among members of the health care team or assigned in part to committees or to an official patient's advocate or hospital ombudsman. I mention these procedures for illustrative purposes only, not to enter into a debate about their respective merits. My point is the importance of having *some* procedures, not *which* should be adopted.

Some procedures of both moral reasoning and moral accountability are important in order to express equal respect, which is perhaps the major reason for requiring patient autonomy in medical decision-making. They should minimize the chances that an adult patient will be treated as a child when in fact he or she is competent to exercise self-determination. Fair and impartial procedures should be designed to increase the likelihood of certain outcomes, because both the outcomes and the procedures themselves express a moral commitment to treat persons as equals. To deprive a person of autonomy without regard for such procedures deepens the affront to dignity by assuming without actually meeting the relevant burden of proof.

However they are designed and implemented, these procedures of accountability will frequently involve nonmedical professionals and laypersons. They express only part of the respect due patients and only one aspect of our conflicting social expectations of medicine. On the one hand, our society cries out for an expansion of medical responsibility to matters formerly handled in other ways. For example, alcoholism, once treated as a social problem, is today assigned to medical professionals. If we accepted the World Health Organization's definition of health ("a state of complete physical, mental, and social well-being"), we would tend to develop an extremely broad, perhaps limitless definition of medical responsibility. In addition to this tendency to "medicalize" more and more areas of social life, there is a tendency to expand concerns within the current definitions and practices of medicine. There are demands that medical professionals should treat the "whole" patient, the patient who has a disease, rather than only the patient's disease. Both this *internal* expansion of medical responsibility and the *external* expansion previously discussed suggest increased professional autonomy.

On the other hand, there are public calls to limit medical responsibility to technical matters and to limit professional autonomy by various procedures designed to ensure patient autonomy.[17] It is difficult to determine which of these social tendencies is dominant and what sort of settlement might be reached between them. On the one hand, society appears to encourage professional autonomy and hence professional paternalism; on the other hand, it appears to encourage patient autonomy by limiting professional responsibility and discretion. Such social conflicts can only exacerbate tensions within medical roles.

The mandate for certain procedures of accountability symbolizes only one segment of our social expectations and only part of what respect for persons involves. I have argued that we should establish practices that acknowledge the moral presumption for patient autonomy and that include procedures of moral reasoning and accountability in order to respect patients as persons. But antipaternalistic policies may be construed in ways other than their proponents and practitioners intend. For example, if we do not intervene to prevent suicides out of respect for patient autonomy, our nonintervention may be seen as expressing the conviction that these deaths do not matter. A policy that affirms "you should care for yourself" may be interpreted as "we don't care for you." "Benign neglect" may be mere indifference or even malevolence. In short, we need practices and procedures

that can indicate care and concern—the attitude of bene-
volence underlying paternalism—even as we try to limit
the refusal to accept or to acquiesce in an individual's
wishes, choices, and actions regarding his or her own
welfare.[18]

Chapter 2

TO LIVE
OR LET DIE

In Edward Bond's play *Bingo: Scenes of Money and Death* a character says, "Only a god or a devil can write in other men's blood and not ask *why* they spilt it and *what* it cost."[1] Never qualifying as gods and only rarely as devils, we have to ask *why* and *at what cost* we allow different classes of patients, such as seriously defective newborns and comatose adults, to die. Part of what it means to be human is to seek warrants for one's conduct and to offer reasons to others. Our humanity can rarely face the spilling of blood without a demand for justification. In addition to the questions *why* and *at what cost,* we are compelled to inquire *how* blood is spilled and *who decides.* These four questions need to be raised in the context of discussions about the care of sick, terminally ill, and dying patients. They are critically important not only for health care providers but also for religious groups and, indeed, for all of us who will probably confront these questions as we make decisions about our own care and the care of relatives. Such decisions may also be made about us. Because of the current philosophical and theological controversy about *how* death is brought about, I shall concentrate first on that question. But before going into the four questions I want to identify our context more precisely.

First, I shall generally avoid using the term "euthanasia." It is not essential and it often confuses the issues because of its widely differing connotations. We tend to decide which cases of killing or allowing to die we find acceptable and then define "euthanasia" to include or exclude those cases, according to what the term "euthanasia" connotes for us.

Second, discussions of ethical issues in death and dying, particularly killing and allowing to die, cover a range of cases from defective newborns to competent adults. I shall try to identify issues that are pertinent to most of these cases and indicate in passing a few special issues that merge in some of them.

Third, we cannot resolve all our dilemmas about how to treat patients by drawing up better criteria for determining death. Of course, if a patient is dead, no further medical care is required. But criteria for determining whether a patient is dead must not be confused with criteria for determining when certain kinds of treatment (e.g., the use of respirators) may be withheld or stopped. Two distinct questions are raised: When is a patient dead? and When is it permissible to withhold treatment so that a living patient may be allowed to die?

HOW IS DEATH BROUGHT ABOUT?

Let us start with the question: How is blood spilled, or death brought about? This question invites distinctions between direct and indirect actions, between killing and allowing to die, and between ordinary and extraordinary means. While these distinctions are especially at home in classic Roman Catholic ethics, they are also affirmed by other religious and secular traditions as well as professional ethical codes. Some commentators dismiss these distinctions as "moral quibbles," others insist that they have a "moral bite." From my own perspective, each distinction is morally important in some settings, largely as a shorthand expression of more complex moral positions.

While the rule of double effect, built on the distinction between direct and indirect intentions and consequences of actions, is often used in debates about legitimate "abortions," it has only limited value in the care of patients. Consider the physician's conflicting duties—not to kill patients and to relieve the pain and suffering of patients. In some situations it might be possible to relieve pain and suffering only by *indirectly* hastening death. Death would be the indirect effect of a legitimate action aimed at the relief of pain, the direct effect. Few people dispute the moral legitimacy of such actions. According to the Ethical and Religious Directives for Catholic Health Facilities, "it is not euthanasia to give a dying person sedatives and analgesics for the alleviation of pain, when such a measure is judged necessary, even though they may deprive the patient of the use of reason, or shorten his life." Nevertheless, the theoretical justification for the rule of double effect is controversial, and the rule itself applies to very few cases.[2]

The second distinction—between killing and allowing to die —is more controversial. The House of Delegates of the American Medical Association in 1973 affirmed this distinction between killing and letting die. It rejected killing as "contrary to that for which the medical profession stands and . . . to the policy of the AMA." But it approved letting patients die in certain cases, such as when the means to prolong life would be extraordinary. Nevertheless, several philosophers and theologians have called this distinction into question. In a widely quoted article in *The New England Journal of Medicine,* James Rachels tries to show that the distinction is not morally relevant. He draws two cases that differ only in that one involves killing and the other involves letting someone die.

> In the first, *Smith* stands to gain a large inheritance if anything should happen to his six-year-old cousin. One evening while the child is taking his bath, Smith breaks into the bathroom and drowns the child, and then arranges things so that it will look like an accident.
> In the second, *Jones* also stands to gain if anything should happen to his six-year-old cousin. Like Smith, Jones sneaks in planning to drown the child in his bath.

However, just as he enters the bathroom Jones sees the child slip and hit his head, and fall face down in the water. Jones is delighted; he stands by, ready to push the child's head back under if it is necessary, but it is not necessary. With only a little thrashing about, the child drowns all by himself, "accidentally," as Jones watches and does nothing.[3]

Smith killed his cousin, whereas Jones allowed his cousin to die. Rachels insists that if killing in itself were worse than letting die, we would say that Smith's act is more reprehensible than Jones's. No doubt we would agree with Rachels that both acts are equally reprehensible because of Smith's and Jones's motives, ends, and what they did. Thus, Rachels argues, the "bare difference" between killing and letting die does not in itself make a "moral difference" and cannot serve to distinguish active and passive euthanasia in the medical context.

Rachels' examples may not be as conclusive as he thinks. Smith's and Jones's vicious motives obscure other features of the case which might be important in other settings. It was wrong for Jones to let his cousin die, because he could and should have saved him. Even if Jones had no other reason, the duty of beneficence (the benefiting of others) requires rescue efforts when they involve only minimal risk or inconvenience and when no one else can undertake them. At the very least, Jones violated a duty of beneficence for a selfish end.

His case throws no light on our dilemmas in the use of biomedical technology. These dilemmas arise precisely because we do not know what constitutes "doing good" for patients in all cases. Let us assume that in many cases physicians and families want to do what is best for their patients and relatives. But they are bewildered. What does it mean to do good, to render care, in these circumstances? Does care require prolonging life for a dying patient who has no hope of recovery or for a patient who will never regain consciousness according to the best medical prognosis? Medical dilemmas are perplexing precisely because physicians and families want to act in the best interests of patients but are unclear about the scope and content of the obligation to care.

Rachels may be right that we should not focus on the "bare difference" between killing and letting die. Even if the bare difference does not show up in every case, even if it is not always morally significant, we may find *religious* and *moral* reasons to affirm the distinction in medical contexts. According to one theological ethicist, we can see the "moral significance" of this distinction only by putting it in the context of the religious stories that gave rise to it.[4] That context includes God's purposes and actions toward his creatures. In that context it makes sense to talk about "letting go," placing patients in God's hands, or entrusting them to God. It is important not to usurp divine prerogatives by killing the patient, but it is also important not to usurp them by desperately struggling to prolong life when the patient is irreversibly dying. Within this religious context, death cannot be viewed as the ultimate enemy; and even if death need not be welcomed, it need not always be opposed. To stop the battle does not mean to abandon the patient or to cease caring for the patient. Optimal care does not always mean maximal treatment. Caring continues even when the patient is allowed to die.

There may be *moral* reasons in addition to specifically religious reasons for affirming the distinction between killing and allowing to die and for prohibiting the former, while permitting the latter in some cases. (It is important to note that even if we defend this distinction between killing and letting die on either religious or moral grounds and exclude killing, we are not committed to saying that all cases of letting die are morally right and even morally better than all cases of killing; that is, many factors other than the *how* question are relevant to an assessment of the act.) Indeed, I do not think the religious context, however important it was in developing the distinction, is a logical presupposition of the distinction; independent moral grounds are sufficient to support it. This distinction between killing and letting die is so interwoven with our understanding of medical care that we cannot remove it without tearing the whole fabric. To authorize physicians to kill patients would so alter the ethos of medicine that a new basis for trust would be necessary.

Sometimes we use the term "trust" ironically, as in Joseph Heller's novel *Something Happened,* when Slocum says of a character: "He knows I drink and lie and whore around a lot, and he therefore feels that he can trust me."[5] Most often, however, trust is the expectation that others will respect certain moral limits. When we trust others, we have confidence that they will act within certain limits toward us (e.g., will not harm us). In the medical context, trust includes the confidence that practitioners will provide personal care, respect us as persons, work for our life and health, and will not harm us intentionally. For the Hippocratic tradition of medical ethics, the physician's first, minimum duty is to do no harm—*primum non nocere.*

This trust is not to be confused with the dependence of the "sick role," although the patient's vulnerability certainly enhances the value of a relationship of trust. Much medical care depends on the patient's trusting response to the physician. While relationships of trust are valued as conditions for other relationships and as means to accomplish other ends, such as successful medical care, they are also valued as ends in themselves. Trust is fragile and, once weakened, is difficult to restore. One Harris poll in the latter part of 1973 discovered that only two of twenty-two institutions were deemed trustworthy by a majority of those questioned. Fifty-seven percent trusted the medical profession, and 52 percent had confidence in local trash collectors! The other institutions, including the police, the press, the church, Congress, and so forth, evoked less confidence.

David Louisell contends that "euthanasia would threaten the patient-physician relationship: confidence might give way to suspicion. . . . Can the physician, historic battler for life, become an affirmative agent of death without jeopardizing the trust of his dependents?"[6] Perhaps trust within medical care does not depend on a prohibition of all killing. But the trust that now characterizes the relationship between patient and physician is based on the medical profession's implicit and explicit commitments to foster life and health. This line of argument stresses the prohibition of killing as one important expression of medical care aimed at the patient's life and health. It is also instrumentally important, for its removal could weaken the constraints on medical practice that make trust possible. At stake is the set of commitments and values that undergird medical care and ground trust.

Although I am sympathetic with this line of argument, it is subject to several objections. First, it is a form of the wedge (exceptions to a law are a dangerous wedge leading to broader exceptions) or the slippery slope (a moral slide may occur if certain restraints are removed) argument which points to what "might" happen. It is appropriate to ask whether we have evidence to think that the terrible consequences would in fact occur. Much would depend on other forces at work in the society—for example, whether we could find other important and enforceable boundaries. But it is also essential to determine whether such an alternative vision of medical and health care is as desirable as our current vision.

Second, one of the strongest arguments for killing some patients directly rather than allowing them to die is the relief of unbearable and uncontrollable pain. Those who offer this argument often appeal to situations outside medicine to show that direct killing is more humane and compassionate—for example, a driver trapped in a burning wreck, or a mortally wounded comrade left on the battlefield as an army retreats.[7] Actually there may be few cases within medical practice where pain cannot be controlled and managed. But even if there are such cases, we have to be careful about trying to build a social or professional ethic on borderline cases. Hard cases may make bad social and professional ethics. It may be morally important to have a rule of practice that prohibits direct killing and authorizes allowing some patients to die in some circumstances even if this rule fails to fit every exceptional case that might be encountered or imagined.

Rather than change this rule of practice, embodied in law and professional codes, to accommodate exceptional cases some theologians argue for acts of conscientious objection or civil disobedience.[8] It is better, they contend, for the rule to remain intact even if physicians and families should sometimes conscientiously disobey it. Most practices also recognize ways to *excuse* certain acts without *justifying* them. For example, persons who have killed suffering relatives have often been found not guilty by reason of temporary insanity. Although these acts of "mercy killing" were not legally justified, they were excused; the agents were not held responsible for them. These ways to accommodate exceptional acts have their own costs which need closer attention.

If this argument is sound, there may be a "right to die," but there is no "right to be killed." While the right to die is a negative right, the right to be killed is a positive right. A negative right is a justified claim to noninterference. If X has a negative right, Y has a duty not to interfere with X's exercise of that right. A positive right, however, is a justified claim to someone's assistance—for example, in suicide or euthanasia. A positive right to be killed would make the physician a tool, and it would probably be deleterious to medical practice in ways that I have already indicated. Our language of "mercy killing" appropriately expresses that no "right" is involved; "mercy" is expressed in actions to which the other has no right.

The third distinction regarding *how* death is brought about is between ordinary and extraordinary medical means. Like the other distinctions, it is an attempt to determine whether an act that results in death is to be counted as killing and especially as culpable killing. In a classic statement by Gerald Kelly, S.J., "Ordinary means are all medicines, treatments, and operations, which offer a reasonable hope of benefit and which can be obtained and used without excessive expense, pain, or other inconvenience. Extraordinary means are all medicines, treatments, and operations, which cannot be obtained or used without excessive expense, pain, or other inconvenience, or which, if used, would not offer a reasonable hope of benefit."[9] Unfortunately, the terms "ordinary" and "extraordinary" are ambiguous. They appear to be shorthand expressions: What is ordinary is required, what is extraordinary is optional. Then it is necessary to determine the *grounds* for holding that a treatment is required or optional. Sometimes the grounds have been found in medical practice: A treatment is required if it is customary, and optional if it is unusual treatment for a particular disease. But these grounds are not adequate, for what is customary treatment for a patient with pneumonia may not be morally required if the patient also suffers from terminal cancer and if the treatment would only prolong the dying process. Most countersuggestions focus on the balance of probable benefits and burdens to the patient. If the treatment has no reasonable prospect of benefiting the patient, it is clearly morally optional. Similarly, if the burdens (e.g., the suffering caused by chemotherapy) outweigh the probable benefits (e.g., extension of life by four to six weeks), the treatment is morally optional. From this standpoint, no single treatment or procedure can be classified as obligatory or optional. For example, the use of a respirator or intravenous feeding may be obligatory or optional, depending on the patient's condition.

Obviously this third distinction regarding *how* death is brought about raises the questions *why* and *who* decides.[10]

WHY ALLOW PATIENTS TO DIE?

A character in Jean Renoir's *The Rules of the Game* says, "You see in this world there is one awful thing, and that is that everyone has his reasons."[11] Yet not all reasons are equally acceptable. The distinction between ordinary and extraordinary suggests that the balance of benefits and burdens is important. But this metaphor of balancing is unhelpful until we know *what* counts as benefits and burdens, *how much* those benefits and burdens are to count, and *whose* benefits and burdens are to be counted. I want to concentrate on the last point: Whose benefits and burdens are relevant? Charles Fried identifies the most important question raised by the publication of policies of withholding or withdrawing life-prolonging measures at the Massachusetts General Hospital and Beth Israel Hospital:

> At whose good are these new statements aimed? Are they aimed at freeing the patient from the tyranny of a technologic (or bureaucratic-professional) imperative to keep alive at all costs, a tyranny that many thinking persons fear as more or less distant menace to their well-being and liberty in their last days? Or are they aimed at freeing society from the burden and expense of caring for a growing multitude of extravagantly demanding moribund persons?[12]

Within a framework of personal care for patients, we should recognize their moral and legal right to refuse treatment. They should have priority in judging their own interests although they depend, in part, on medical judgments too. The hard cases involve patients who cannot make decisions or express their wishes—for example, a comatose adult or a defective newborn. In these cases, decisions should be made only in terms of the patient's best interest. Although the competent patient may legitimately consider whether the proposed treatment is excessively burdensome to others in view of the benefit to be expected, that consideration should not be the basis of others' decisions about the patient's care. To allow other parties to make decisions about the care on grounds other than the patient's own interests is to open the door to serious social abuse and decline of trust.

In contrast to my approach, some commentators argue that we should use standards of social benefit and harm to make life-death decisions. For example, Raymond Duff reported that 14 percent of 299 consecutive deaths over thirty months at Yale–New Haven's Special-Care Nursery resulted from decisions to withhold or withdraw treatment. Duff holds that there

is a "family commons," consisting of limited, private resources
on which families depend to survive and function. He insists
that we should allow families to refuse treatment for defective
newborns who would put great strain on their emotional and
financial resources: "There are times . . . when one must decide
between the well-being of the unfortunate and that of others
in competition for limited resources. By direct or proxy decision, it may be reasonable at times to make a tragic choice of
neglect, even death, for one in order to protect others."[13]

The reasons that Duff adduces are not weighty enough to my
mind to justify killing defective newborns or allowing them to
die. Christians and others have appealed to various criteria to
justify the use of lethal force against others; these criteria,
invoked in self-defense and war, include just cause, last resort,
and proportionality.[14] By these criteria, a defective newborn's
threat to the "family commons" is not sufficient to justify killing it or allowing it to die. Obviously there are alternative
means, such as putting the infant in an institution or up for
adoption.

To restrict the reasons for withholding or withdrawing treatment to the patient's own interests may appear unduly harsh
to families faced with the prospect of caring for a seriously
defective newborn who needs an operation to survive. In such
cases, society should assume a greater burden by providing
financial and other support services to care for this patient.

Although decisions about defective newborns and incompetent adults should rest exclusively on their own interests and
not on the interests of others, there may be significant differences between these cases. The incompetent adult has a past,
a history, in the light of which we could say that "he or she
would not want to live under these conditions." A judgment
about that patient's best interest draws on his or her biography.
Further treatment may be deemed useless or without sufficient
benefit to that person. How that person's biography, with its
values and aspirations, should be reconstructed, and by whom,
may not be easy to determine. The New Jersey Supreme Court

refused to rely on Karen Ann Quinlan's previous comments to her friends that she would want to die under such conditions. A "living will," properly executed in states that authorize such wills, would have more weight.[15]

In cases involving defective newborns, we might say that no "reasonable" person would want to be kept alive under those circumstances. Attempts to formulate satisfactory criteria of "quality of life" or "meaningful life" have been notoriously vague and inconclusive. One possible starting point is Richard McCormick's proposal that we consider "the potential for human relationships."[16] Where this potential is totally lacking, the obligation to care does not require treatment.

Standards of "quality of life" or "meaningful life" require protection from insidious judgments of social worth. Marc Lappé contends that our judgments of quality of life tend to reflect the requirements and aspirations of the American ethic. He notes that we are inclined to define quality of life in terms of productivity, and physicians are inclined to treat patients with neurological and mental difficulties less vigorously than patients with physical difficulties.[17] Joseph Fletcher's criteria of "humanhood" are also suspect because they are framed in terms of his standard of utility or social worth, i.e., the individual's potential contribution to society.[18] In addition, they are maximal. They define not merely the *boundaries* but also the *ideal* of humanhood. One criterion, for example, is the balance of rationality and feeling.

According to Paul Ramsey, even to consider "quality of life" is dangerous. It is to shift the question from whether *treatments* are beneficial to patients to whether patients' *lives* are beneficial to themselves. The latter question, he contends, opens the door to active, involuntary euthanasia.[19] Perhaps this danger is evident in the case of Earle Spring, a seventy-eight-year-old man who suffered from senility and chronic kidney failure. Because of his senility he was in a nursing home, and because of his chronic kidney failure, he required dialysis. Although he indicated to nurses that he did not want to die, his wife and son sought court approval to remove him from dialysis so that he could die. The Massachusetts Supreme Court approved this request, a month after his death. As George Annas suggests, "The case seems to have been decided on quality-of-life considerations," although the court did not explicitly invoke them.[20]

The difficulties and dangers are evident. Perhaps the language of "quality of life" or "meaningful life" is too loose and vague, too susceptible to corruption by judgments of social worth, and too easily directed against the senile and mentally retarded. At the very least, such slogans should be replaced by "the patient's best interest." Such a shift will not resolve all difficulties or avoid all risks, for the criteria of "the patient's best interest" are by no means evident. Nor is it clear how loudly we should applaud recent efforts to develop and enforce public definitions of the patient's interest. Although these efforts appear to provide more protection for incompetent patients by reducing discretion, they too have their costs. In the long run, their impact may be more negative for the mentally retarded, for example, than earlier policies that allowed familial and medical discretion.

WHO DECIDES?

Who decides, or should decide, that allowing a patient to die is in that patient's best interest? First, the competent patient in consultation with the physician. Determination that the treatment is extraordinary involves both medical and value judgments. Only the physician can determine the chances of success of a particular treatment, but only the patient can determine whether the course of action is satisfactory. But even the patient's right to refuse treatment is not absolute. Although it is not morally permissible to kill patients or to let patients die for the sake of others, it is sometimes justifiable to keep them alive even against their wishes for the sake of others (e.g., a child's need for a mother). And "weak" paternalistic interferences with a patient's decisions are sometimes justified. They must, however, meet a heavy burden of proof.

If the patient is incompetent and cannot make decisions, who should decide? The family? physicians? hospital committees? courts? All these groups have been recommended as the primary decision makers for incompetent patients. If familiarity with the formerly competent patient and his or her values is important, the family may be recommended. If technical expertise is valued, physicians and other health care professionals may be proposed. If fairness and impartiality are to be stressed, the courts may be appropriate.

Paul Ramsey, for example, holds that judgments about whether and which treatment ought to be provided really depend on objective "medical indications." Physicians as agents, he argues, should make such decisions about patients in the context of their own commitment to care for and preserve life rather than to serve patients' wishes. The physicians' decisions should be based on medical factors that are objective even though they cannot be infallibly determined. Even for conscious, competent patients, Ramsey does not emphasize a right of refusal, but rather a right to "participate" in medical decisions that affect them.[21] Because the primary factors are medical rather than valuational, medical personnel have priority in decisions regarding incompetent patients.

But if the question of whether (and which) treatment ought to be provided depends on an evaluation of the patient's condition, broadly conceived to include the patient's interests, the family should have priority in decision-making because of presumed familiarity with and presumed identification with the patient's values. And they should have priority in decisions about a defective newborn because of their presumed interest in the child's welfare. Insofar as the decisions are valuative, there is no reason to remove them from the family. But this priority of the family is not final. If physicians and other health care professionals believe that a familial decision to terminate treatment is against a patient's best interest, they should try to persuade the members of the family to change their minds. If necessary, the health care professionals should appeal to the courts to authorize treatment. They do not merely provide information and withdraw, acquiescing in familial decision which they believe violates the patient's interests. They remain moral agents rather than mere technicians.

Most so-called Ethics Committees as mandated by the New Jersey Supreme Court in the famous Karen Ann Quinlan case really serve only to verify medical judgments (e.g., that there is little chance that the patient will regain cognitive, sapient life) rather than to make ethical judgments. If the function of the committees is to make ethical judgments, they do not appear to be necessary and may only serve to diffuse responsibility.

AT WHAT COST?

Finally, what would be the bad consequences or "cost" of implementing a practice of allowing patients to die? As the narrator of John Updike's novel *Couples* suggests after Foxy's abortion, "Death, once invited in, leaves his muddy bootprints everywhere."[22] If we accept a policy of ending life even under the conditions I have mentioned (i.e., letting die, not killing, only in the patient's interest after rebutting a presumption that the patient would want to live), would we then be able to limit the spilling of blood to cases that seem legitimate? Some point to the Holocaust and other horrors to indicate where we will end up if we fail to blunt the edge of the wedge or to stay off the slippery slope.

These wedge or slippery slope arguments may take one of two forms. One version focuses on the moral reasoning behind acts and claims that if the reasoning is unsound, there will be no line between the conduct we allow and the conduct we want to avoid. This version of the wedge argument may hold, for instance, that to justify allowing to die is also to justify killing, because there is no morally significant distinction between them.

The other version holds that forces in society make a "moral slide" probable and perhaps even inevitable if we remove certain restraints. Even if our moral reasoning is sound, so that logically we can distinguish two sorts of cases, we cannot count on people to draw these distinctions in practice. Various psychological or sociological factors will lead us into a moral quagmire if we fail to maintain certain limits. The first version appeals to the logic of moral reasoning, the second to empirical analysis.

Although such arguments are often drawn to support indefensible positions, they cannot be dismissed. Sometimes they apply. For example, I invoked them in my defense of prohibiting killing in medical care and, indirectly, in my defense of restricting the range of reasons for allowing a patient to die. I appealed to the probable consequences, such as abuse and decline of trust, if we accepted a policy of killing patients or including familial or social interests along with the patient's interests.

Several major fears invite the wedge or slippery slope arguments even against policies that I have endorsed. One fear concerns *why* we allow patients to die: a possible or probable slide from the patient's interests to familial or social interests. A second fear concerns *who* decides: a possible or probable slide from voluntary (requested or accepted by the patient) or nonvoluntary (without the patient's will which cannot be known) to involuntary (against the patient's express wishes). A third fear focuses on *how* death is brought about: a possible or probable slide from passive to active, or from letting die to killing.

It is possible to avoid the implications of either version of the wedge or slippery slope argument if we carefully construct substantive and procedural standards along the lines suggested above. Let me reemphasize some of the criteria. First, there should be a presumption in favor of prolonging life; this should be our starting point. Second, this presumption may be rebutted when the patient, in consultation with physicians, decides that the proposed treatment is not acceptable. While the patient should have the right to make this decision, his or her refusal of treatment may sometimes be overridden on weak paternalistic grounds, as indicated in Chapter 1. Third, when the patient lacks the capacity to decide, the decision may be made by an authorized representative of the patient's interests, usually the family, in consultation with physicians whose medical assessments are indispensable. The only acceptable reason for allowing a patient to die, when the decision is not made by the patient, is the patient's best interest. When physicians and other health care professionals believe that the family's decision is not in the patient's best interest, they should seek to overrule it. Fourth, we should prohibit killing but authorize allowing to die in cases that meet the above conditions.

If we structure our practice along these lines, if we accept these answers to *who* may end life and *why* and *how* life may be ended, any social cost will probably be negligible. And if we continue to test our practice with all four questions—*how, who, why,* and *at what cost*—we may be able to resist the temptation to play the role of a god or a devil.[23]

Chapter 3

HUMAN SUBJECTS
IN RESEARCH

Moral concern about the use of human subjects in research has been widespread since the horrendous Nazi experiments came to light. Various medical and legal codes, such as the Nuremberg Code and the Declaration of Helsinki, offer principles and guidelines about what may be done to research subjects for the sake of scientific progress.[1] Concern about this issue has fluctuated in the United States, usually rising as news breaks about "big bang" or "neon light" cases. In 1966, *The New England Journal of Medicine* published Henry Beecher's article on "Ethics and Clinical Research," which documented many cases of unethical or questionable research involving human subjects.[2] In the early 1970s, the Tuskegee study in which many syphilitic black men were left untreated without their consent in order to trace the natural history of syphilis provoked outrage.[3] Indeed, reaction to this Tuskegee study and to the use of fetuses for research after the Supreme Court in 1973 overturned restrictive abortion laws was a major reason that Congress created the National Commission for the Protection of Human Subjects of Biomedical and Behavioral Research. Its mandate, in part, was to "conduct a comprehensive investigation and study to identify the *basic ethical principles* which should underlie the conduct of biomedical and behavioral research involving human subjects" (Public Law 93–

348). This Commission, appointed in December 1974, recommended guidelines for research involving fetuses, children, prisoners, and the institutionalized mentally infirm. Rarely has there been as much ethical analysis in the formation of policy.

While the National Commission's work is perhaps the most dramatic example of ethical reflection on research involving human subjects, discussions abound in various forums and publications. Yet tensions persist and even increase, in part because of misunderstanding and in part because of fundamental ethical disagreements. Much of the confusion probably stems from the failure by many parties to the debate to identify the real issues. The dilemmas are often wrongly posed. "Moral values versus scientific progress" is one example of such a fundamentally misleading formulation. It implies that the medical and biological sciences operate in opposition to human moral values. While that formulation may be accurate in some cases, it fails to identify the most important ethical questions. There are moral dilemmas in research involving human subjects because our moral principles cross one another. Because we cannot always realize all the relevant moral principles and values, we face dilemmas and have to determine which principles and values should take priority. Unavoidable dilemmas result from conflicts between individual rights and social needs, between respect for the integrity of the individual and furthering the welfare of groups. Morality is not simply on one side or the other.

To help sort out the issues, I shall analyze some models of ethical reflection on research involving human subjects. I shall argue for a pluralist model and delineate the criteria that this model requires. Then I shall consider what the standard of voluntary, informed consent implies for certain difficult areas in research and whether society has a duty to compensate injured research subjects.

Models of Ethical Reflection

The first model is *consequentialist.* [4] It emphasizes the values of scientific knowledge: the conquest of numerous diseases, the increase in life expectancy, and the improved quality of life. The basic ethical design of this model is balancing benefits against risks. The language of rights is generally avoided, because rights cannot be quantified and calculated. Rights are sometimes translated into interests and needs so that they can be balanced and subjected to trade-offs. Thus the emphasis in the consequentialist model is not on the rights, liberty, and autonomy of the human subject but is on the autonomy of the biomedical profession, since only the researchers have the knowledge to determine the research's risk-benefit ratio. The major imperative of the consequentialist model is, "Achieve good." Some extreme versions of this model imply that ends justify means, perhaps even to the extent expressed by the late labor organizer, Saul Alinsky, who held that those who worry about means in relation to ends usually wind up on their ends with no means at all.

Over against this consequentialist model is the *deontological* model of ethical reflection. For this model, some acts, attitudes, and policies are right apart from their effects or consequences. It emphasizes individual rights that are not subject to balancing in a cost-benefit or harm-benefit model. The deontological model presents such moral rules as "Do not use human subjects without their informed consent." Such a rule is itself grounded in more fundamental values, such as autonomy, self-determination, and the right of individuals to be treated as ends. In this perspective, to act against a person's wishes or without the person's consent is to treat that person as a means to some private or social good. Such acts violate that person's fundamental rights. In this model the freedom of the subject, not of the biomedical professions, is critical. When a person becomes a subject in human research, that person is more than a subject. Such a person is a participant, a coadventurer, a collaborator in research, and is to be treated as such.[5]

Defenders of the deontological model admit that respecting these rights may well limit some scientific research or make it more costly. As Charles Fried concedes, rights constrain and limit the pursuit of social goods; and all may not work out for the best, because this is not the best of all possible worlds.[6] More graphically, a right that doesn't stick in the spokes of someone's wheels is no right at all. Rights are what Ronald Dworkin has called "political trumps."[7] The ethical imperative for the deontological model is, "Violate no rights."

The third model can be called a *pluralist* model. It includes both consequentialist and deontological themes. It recognizes independent rights and gives them considerable weight, but it also recognizes the importance of consequences. It is implicit in Paul Ramsey's contention that the ends justify the means, but not all means.[8] I think that this model is closer to the way we actually think and reason in this area. Criteria that operate in the pluralist model apply to some extent in other areas, such as the justification of war. The reason is simple: the same or analogous criteria are used whenever we encounter situations that involve conflicting values, duties, or obligations.

The starting point of the pluralist model is a presumption that can be overridden under some circumstances. This presumption is that we should not subject anyone to research. It is important to distinguish therapeutic and nontherapeutic research, though other terms might be preferable. Nontherapeutic research is designed to generate knowledge, not to benefit the subjects who participate in it. Therapeutic research, however, is designed to generate knowledge and to benefit sick patient-subjects. An example of nontherapeutic research would be the testing of drugs on normal subjects in order to determine safety and toxicity. Testing such drugs on sick patients who may benefit from the drugs would be therapeutic research. Both nontherapeutic and therapeutic research should be distinguished from regular or innovative therapy designed to benefit the patient without any plan to produce generaliz-able knowledge.

Because a cardinal principle of biomedical ethics is, "Do no harm," there is a presumption against both nontherapeutic and therapeutic research. In the former, normal persons are put at risk for the sake of others; in the latter, sick persons are put at risk for the sake of others. But this presumption is rebuttable, and the model explains *when* it is rebuttable.

CRITERIA OF ETHICALLY JUSTIFIED RESEARCH

First, there should be a *morally important reason* for the research. Some ends are moral in that their pursuit is not im-moral; some are moral in that their pursuit is morally required; and some are moral in that their pursuit is praiseworthy though not mandatory. Stopping a plague might be morally required. Some improvements in the human condition might be moral in one of the other two senses. It is not sufficient to evaluate research as a whole, for it is also necessary to evaluate each particular research proposal in terms of its aims.

Second, there should be a *reasonable prospect* that the research will generate the knowledge that is sought. This condition focuses on the research design. Moral evaluation cannot be separated from scientific evaluation: for if the research design is faulty, the research is unlikely to be productive. To proceed is both bad ethics and bad science. As the Nuremberg Code indicates, "the experiment should be so designed and based on the results of animal experimentation and a knowledge of the natural history of the disease or other problem under study that the anticipated results will justify the performance of the experiment."

Third, the use of human subjects in this research should be a matter of *last resort;* their use should be *necessary.* Such use of human subjects must be preceded by other studies, including animal experimentation. Then, we must still need to know how human beings respond before it is justified to use them in research. The Nuremberg Code holds that "the experiment should be such as to yield fruitful results for the good of society, *unprocurable by other methods or means of study.*" It may be appropriate, for instance, to ask whether Stanley Milgram's famous studies of obedience were really necessary. Milgram established that 65 percent of his subjects were willing to inflict what they thought was intense physical pain on other persons through electrical shocks as part of what they believed to be a learning experiment.[9] Perhaps we are too beguiled by the scientific model to be satisfied with other kinds of evidence. Moral questions thus might be raised not only about the experiment's design, but also about its necessity and its importance.

A new drug, ara-A, was known to be useful in treating herpes and to have no demonstrable hepatic, renal, or hematologic toxicity. A question remained, Would it be useful in treating herpes simplex encephalitis, which has a mortality rate of approximately 70 percent? In a clinical trial, some patient-subjects with the disease received the experimental drug, ara-A; others received standard treatment. But is it necessary to give standard treatment when that treatment is known to be ineffective, when the risk is death, and when the experimental treatment has already been shown not to be toxic? Historical controls—that is, what was known about the mortality rate with standard treatment—would probably have been sufficient. In the controlled trial, seven of the ten patients who received the standard treatment died, and only two recovered to lead reasonably normal lives. Of the eighteen patients who received ara-A, seven recovered to lead reasonably normal lives, while the other six had serious brain or nerve damage. The experiment was eventually stopped, and all patients received ara-A.[10]

Fourth, the research should meet the principle of *proportionality.* This principle involves risk-benefit analysis. As Department of Health, Education, and Welfare guidelines (1978) indicate, a review must be conducted to determine whether "the risks to the subject are so outweighed by the sum of the benefit to the subject and the importance of the knowledge to be gained as to warrant a decision to allow the subject to accept these risks."[11] In addition to the first criterion, which had to do with the value of the end that is sought, this criterion adds the consideration of risks in comparison to the benefits—an indispensable but difficult task. "The degree of risk to be taken should never exceed that determined by the humanitarian importance of the problem to be solved by the experiment." (Nuremberg Code.)

Fifth, the research must have the subject's *voluntary* and *informed consent* to participate.

These first five criteria are indispensable considerations from a moral standpoint.[12] Each of them must be met in order for research involving human subjects to be ethically justified. It is important to identify a sixth standard: Are the benefits and burdens of research fairly and equitably distributed among the population? This standard does not identify a necessary condition for any particular research project. Rather, it applies to the whole range of research projects in a society; it focuses on policies and patterns in the selection of subjects. To be sure, any particular research project may be unjustified because of its selection of subjects, but to locate a project in a hospital that serves the poor and underprivileged may not be unfair if the burdens and risks of research are generally distributed in a fair way throughout the society. Exploitation is prohibited.

Hans Jonas has proposed a "principle of identification" for recruiting subjects for biomedical research: We should select participants who can identify with the goals and purposes of the research and thus become partners and coadventurers with the researchers. Obviously this principle suggests initial recruitment within the scientific community. But then, Jonas says, "we should look for additional subjects where a maximum of identification, understanding, and spontaneity can be expected—that is, among the most highly motivated, the most highly educated, and the least 'captive' members of the community." Following a descending order of permissibility, Jonas holds that "the poorer in knowledge, motivation and freedom of decision (and that, alas, means the more readily available in terms of numbers and possible manipulation), the more sparingly and indeed reluctantly should the reservoir be used, and the more compelling must therefore become the countervailing justification."[13] In contrast to this standard, we tend in practice to take advantage of the weak and powerless, the poor and uneducated, the imprisoned and institutionalized, and the patients on the ward. Why? Largely as a matter of convenience rather than scientific necessity. It is important to ask what this selection of subjects symbolizes and expresses about our society, its moral qualities and its convictions.

Finally, we need to establish and maintain procedures to ensure that these criteria are met. The cliché about physicians "playing God" needs to have its point sharpened. It refers less, I think, to medicine's great power and more to medicine's lack of accountability in some areas: "Being God," after all, means "never having to say you're sorry." It is not sufficient, however, simply to rely on the virtue of the researcher. We need ways to ensure the accountability of researchers, such as peer review mechanisms and institutional review boards. Important though these procedures are, particularly for applying the first four criteria, they do not ensure the quality of consent sought by investigators and actually given by subjects in research. It is important to know whether a particular subject has actually understood the information given before consenting to participate. Because signed consent forms do not always indicate understanding or voluntariness, we need to develop mechanisms and procedures to ensure that the consent of subjects is informed and free.

INFORMED CONSENT

Why is informed consent important? What does it involve? What does it imply for some problem areas? Many grounds support the requirement of informed consent. The deontological model emphasizes a person's right to determine the use of his or her body. The language of integrity, self-determination, autonomy, and privacy invokes relevant moral and legal considerations. Without this standard of informed consent, the subject is only a tool in the hands of the investigator rather than a participant in a collaborative enterprise. It is important to note that consent is different from approval. We may approve all sorts of actions by others without consenting to them. Consent is a right-creating action; it creates rights in others.

As applied to *competent* persons, the consent standard has two main elements. The first is information. The subject must be informed before he or she can give consent. Many studies of consent reveal misconceptions and misunderstandings on the part of subjects. Even a few minutes after consenting to participate in research, the subject may give little evidence of having received and understood the relevant information.[14] The goal of complete information and complete comprehension is an ideal that cannot be realized, at least in most cases. As a result, most legal and ethical commentators call for a "reasonable man" standard ("reasonable person," of course, but the law hasn't caught up with our current changes in language). I quote from one court case: "The subject of medical experimentation is entitled to a full and frank disclosure of all the facts, probabilities, and opinions which a reasonable man might be expected to consider before giving his consent."[15]

Regarding the sort of information that should be expected, DHEW guidelines (1978) list the following: "(1) a fair explanation of the procedures to be followed, and their purposes, including identification of any procedures which are experimental; (2) a description of any attendant discomforts and risks reasonably to be expected; (3) a description of any benefits reasonably to be expected; (4) a disclosure of any appropriate alternative procedures that might be advantageous for the subject; (5) an offer to answer any inquiries concerning the procedures; and (6) an instruction that the person is free to withdraw his consent and discontinue participation in the project or activity at any time without prejudice to the subject."

The second condition for valid consent is *voluntariness.* The consent must be voluntary—that is, uncoerced. The Nuremberg code of ethics in medical research holds that "the person involved should have legal capacity to give consent; should be so situated as to be able to exercise free power of choice, without the intervention of any element of force, fraud, deceit, duress, overreaching, or other ulterior form of constraint or coercion." This voluntary consent, of course, may involve the acceptance of risk. But it is not enough to say that the experiment can go forward, whatever the degree of risk, if the subject is willing to accept it. All the criteria must be met, including the risk-benefit ratio. The Nuremberg Code says, for instance, that "no experiment should be conducted where there is an *a priori* reason to believe that death or disabling injury will occur." And that standard would apply even in those cases where the person is willing to consent.

Perhaps we should refuse to accept some voluntary risk-taking by some persons in some settings. In his classic essay *On Liberty,* John Stuart Mill held that by and large we may restrict the activity of people and interfere with their liberty only when there is some harm, or threat of harm, to others. But he recognized one paternalistic exception. We should, he said, prevent a person from selling himself into slavery for his own good and future liberty.[16] The consent of the victim should not eliminate our concern for the risk-benefit ratio. It is true that we allow persons to accept risks for themselves all the time—for example, in mountain climbing, skydiving, and other risky sports. In most instances we are inclined to avoid paternalistic legislation. So why not let persons take any risks they are willing to accept in research? The answer is that it is one matter for people to accept certain risks for themselves; it is another matter for a specialized profession, acting on behalf of the entire society, to impose those risks on individuals even when those individuals are willing to accept them. The danger of exploitation is too great.

Too often, informed consent is treated as though it were the only relevant standard for evaluating research. It is only one among several indispensable standards. Indeed, it should not be the first one identified and discussed. Informed consent should be invoked only after other important matters have been examined—the value of the research, the risk-benefit ratio, etc. To concentrate on informed consent may distort the other, prior ethical requirements for research involving human subjects. Nevertheless, one reason for its prominence in contemporary debates is that it authorizes the researcher to proceed with this subject. Even when the other conditions are met, if voluntary and informed consent (or proxy consent) cannot be secured, the research cannot morally proceed.

HARD CASES FOR THE CONSENT REQUIREMENT

Is the requirement to get voluntary, informed consent absolute and unconditional? I think it is virtually without exception. Let me pose a possible exception. A country might conceivably confront a terrible rampant disease that could not be controlled by existing procedures. In such a situation, it might be necessary to draft some people to participate in research. Suppose that the disease in question is so bad and so uncontrollable that the community's very survival appears to be threatened. In such a case there would probably be enough volunteers to enable the necessary research to proceed regardless of the danger. But if we assume that we could not get enough voluntary subjects in the face of this clear and present danger, we might justifiably implement a draft. Of course, there is an analogy to the military draft involving coercion and compulsion. Such a measure would be justified only if there were clearly no other choice, if all other options had been exhausted, and if the community's very survival were threatened. Even these conditions would not justify all means. They would not justify deception, trickery, kidnapping, or other forms of coercion to obtain participants. They would only justify a duly authorized draft, totally aboveboard, with some fair way of imposing the additional burdens of communal existence on some and not on others.

Is there a cogent argument for a draft under *nonemergency* circumstances? Many philosophers and theologians contend that research is desirable but optional because the goal of scientific progress is desirable but optional. Participation in research thus is praiseworthy but not obligatory. Conscription of subjects could be justified not in order to realize good but in order to avoid evil—the disaster for the community. However, at least one moral theologian, Richard McCormick, S.J., holds a stronger view of scientific progress and our minimal social duties.[17] Where others will probably benefit from research, and our participation in research is at "no cost or minimal cost to ourselves," we have a duty of social justice, not only charity, to participate. What are the grounds of this "ought," this duty of social justice? The main ground appears to be our membership in the human community, our interdependence as human beings. McCormick also suggests the principle of fair play—we have benefited from the fruits of medical research in which others have participated, and we now have a duty to take our turn—and the principle of gratitude. Nevertheless, he hesitates to call for a draft, preferring instead consensual community wherever possible. His conclusion is properly qualified, perhaps even to the point of authorizing a draft only in a national emergency: "If, however, not enough volunteers are available for minimal risk experimentation and the research seems of *overriding importance to the public health,* it would not be unjust of the government to recruit experimental subjects." He fails to see, however, that a true national emergency might justify conscription for research involving more than minimal risk, just as military service in wartime involves more than minimal risk. Short of such an emergency, conscription does not appear to be justified, even for low or minimal risk research.

One of the most controversial applications of the principle of respect for persons and its derived rule of voluntary, informed consent is to *prisoners*. Involved in research mainly since World War II (when they were used for antimalarial and other studies as part of the war effort), prisoners have often been used in drug tests. A few years ago it was estimated that more than 85 percent of phase I drug tests (to determine effects, especially toxicity, and safe dosage range in humans) in the United States involved prisoners. Obviously phase I drug tests are the most risky, since phase II determines the effectiveness of the drug and phase III determines the ideal dosage. Prisoners are generally healthy, ambulatory, and mentally competent; they constitute a relatively homogeneous population. They are available for long periods of time for follow-up, and their conditions can be controlled and monitored (e.g., diet and access to other drugs). In addition, their participation costs less than that of normal volunteers. Nevertheless, prisoners are rarely used as research subjects except in the United States.

Critics of the use of prisoners as research subjects insist that even when information is adequate, voluntariness is absent and coercion prevails. Such a claim needs careful scrutiny. First, it is necessary to consider why prisoners participate in research. Studies of research subjects in prison indicate that the three major motivations are financial reimbursement, service to others and to society, and personal advantages such as physical examinations, relaxation, and improved environment.[18] Many of these reasons depend on the prison setting. But is participation for financial reimbursement "involuntary" or "coerced"? Not necessarily, for it depends on the setting of the consent. Critics often insist that prisons as total institutions are inherently coercive: "The state exercises total control over every moment of the prisoner's life. The state tells the prisoner how he must live, when to sleep, when to get up, when to eat, what to eat, what to do and when to do it—all adding up to the most oppressive coercive institution that we have in our society."[19] In such an environment, critics contend, voluntary consent is impossible.

Such a claim is too sweeping.[20] Whether prisoners can give voluntary consent to participate in research depends greatly on the particular prison environment, the type of prison (e.g., whether minimum or maximum security), alternatives to participation in research, procedures and mechanisms to ensure the voluntariness of consent, outside supervision and monitoring, public scrutiny, and even the type of research. Prisoners themselves think that their consent (or refusal) is voluntary. In one major study of four prisons, about 90 percent of the subjects indicated that they would be willing to participate in future experiments.[21] While such statements are significant, they may not be decisive, largely because the issue is not only one of respect for persons and their consent. An equally important issue is the distribution of benefits and burdens of research, my sixth standard of justice.

When the pattern of phase I drug tests over a period of time is considered, it appears that prisoners have borne a disproportionate share of the burdens and risks of this type of research. Society has taken advantage of their availability and their conditions, not, in most cases, by failing to get their voluntary consent but by asking them to participate rather than asking others. We have taken advantage of a captive population from social classes that have received fewer benefits from scientific research, such as improved medical care. What is right for society in this matter may not be what prisoners want. For example, prisoners have opposed the Food and Drug Administration ban, effective June 1, 1981, on the use of prisoners in drug and other medical research unrelated to the health problems of incarcerated persons as a class.[22] The National Commission's conclusion is sound: "Should coercions be lessened and more equitable systems for the sharing of burdens and benefits be devised, respect for persons and concern for justice would suggest that prisoners not be deprived of the opportunity to participate in research."[23]

If prisoners pose special questions about the voluntariness of consent, patients in *controlled clinical trials* pose special questions about disclosure of information, another element of informed consent. Consistent with his principle of identification, Hans Jonas argues that patients are particularly vulnerable and should not be used as research subjects if nonpatients would suffice; in any event, they should be used only in research on the disease(s) from which they suffer.[24] Of course, it is necessary to use patients in order to determine whether a particular treatment for a disease is effective. And, many researchers argue, controlled clinical trials are important, perhaps even essential, to make sure that an observed effect, such as reduced mortality from a disease, really results from a particular treatment, not from some other variables overlooked by the researcher. In a randomized clinical trial, patients are not matched for variables but are randomly assigned to different therapies or placebos; randomization is used to prevent distortion of the study by other variables. Randomized clinical trials (RCTs) are thus preferred to observational or retrospective studies because they appear to offer more certain knowledge. Yet, as we saw in the discussion of ara-A, RCTs are not always necessary; historical controls are sometimes adequate.

What should patient-subjects in RCTs be told at the outset of the trial, as the trial develops, and when they enroll after the trial has been under way for some time? In addition to all the information provided to any subject in research, information about the *method* of allocation of the experimental treatment, standard treatment, and placebo should be provided. Even though it is widely held that RCTs should not be conducted unless researchers are uncertain about the treatments and, some insist, believe that they are "equal," the method of allocating treatments should be disclosed. It is not a matter of indifference to a reasonable person that what he or she receives will be determined randomly. Recently in Denmark a randomized clinical trial was conducted to assess the value of intestinal bypass in the treatment of gross obesity. One hundred and thirty patients received surgery and were compared with sixty-six nonsurgically treated patients. No one who underwent surgery died, and these patient-subjects had "a better improvement in quality of life and a higher degree of patient satisfaction" despite the fact that complications from the operation were "common and occasionally severe." The participants did not give informed consent to participate in the research, for relevant information was withheld and deception was used. The researchers report: "We did not ask for informed consent for randomisation. Patients allocated to medical treatment were told that surgery had to be postponed for an undetermined period primarily because liver-biopsy findings showed fatty infiltration. . . . After randomisation all patients were seen frequently for 36 months; thereafter the individual departments were free to choose type of treatment."[25] This deception was not ethically justified.

The patient-subject can give informed consent even without knowing *what* he or she will receive. Incomplete disclosure is different from deception. Suppose that the patient is asked to participate in a clinical trial that is double-blind: neither the patient-subjects nor the physician-investigators can know who receives what. As long as this information is provided and the patient understands the procedure (as well as the other relevant matters), his or her consent is valid. In addition, it may be useful to have a "surrogate consent system" to test, not to replace, the consent of the participants.[26]

Other information is also morally required, such as role relations that might involve conflicts of interest (e.g., when the same person is both physician and investigator in relation to the same patient) and procedures and mechanisms for early termination of the trial if one treatment proves to be safer or more effective. The latter are particularly important in double-blind trials.

Consent to participate in research is an ongoing process, not a single event. Morally and legally, the patient-subject continues to give consent and may withdraw from the research project at any time for any reason. But then the question emerges: What should patient-subjects be told while the trial is in progress? Should they be told about trends even before the evidence is statistically significant? Such information would enable them to exercise their right to continue or to withdraw more intelligently, but would, in many instances, jeopardize the trial itself. Not disclosing such information in the course of the trial can be morally justified only if patient-subjects understood and consented to this nondisclosure at the outset, if confidentiality of the data remains important and even necessary, and if adequate safeguards exist to protect the patient-subjects.

Another difficult case is the patient-subject who enters a trial that has been under way for some time. Since some trends have emerged, is it proper to tell this new patient-subject what was true at the outset: "We don't know which is better"? This new entrant should receive all the information provided at the outset and should be told, if it is true, that statistical significance has not been reached. If the newcomer is not satisfied and refuses to participate without more information, that is the end of the matter. No deception is morally permissible in this setting. Obviously, the late entrant is asked to trust the investigator, the Institutional Review Board, and the Data and Safety Monitoring Committee, but his or her trust is no greater than what is required of the first patient-subject who still remains in the study. Some trust, as confidence in and reliance upon others, is essential in this setting.

In short, there is a moral presumption for providing all the information that a reasonable person would want and all that this particular person wants. It is a conclusive presumption in that deception is ruled out; it is a rebuttable presumption in that some information (e.g., about the treatment received and emerging trends) may be withheld, or only partially disclosed, (*a*) if the patient-subject consents to this arrangement, (*b*) if nondisclosure is deemed necessary (not merely useful), and (*c*) if adequate protective mechanisms or procedures are in place.

When we are uncertain about substantive ethical matters, we frequently resort to procedures, particularly procedures that can create *moral distance.* This is done by diffusing responsibility (e.g., a committee) or by differentiating roles (e.g., X does this, Y does that, but no one is responsible for the whole). Several examples occur in clinical trials. First, the double-blind design is important not only for scientific reasons but also because it creates "ethical blindness." I do not intend this phrase to be pejorative; it is appropriate because neither the physician-investigator nor the patient-subject knows which treatment is given. Second, some discussants of clinical trials have also proposed that we differentiate roles so that physicians do not use their own patients in research.[27] A person can be both an investigator and a clinician but should not assume both roles for the same patient-subject, just as the physician who proposes to transplant a kidney from A to B should not determine when A is dead. Third, in double-blind studies, another procedure creates some ethical distance: the Data and Safety Monitoring Committee. According to the National Institutes of Health, its function is essentially technical and usually only advisory (e.g., to a higher policy committee or to the local Institutional Review Board that approves the research); it considers the data emerging from the trial and determines whether patient-subjects are harmed and whether trends are statistically significant. This arrangement relocates but does not resolve the critical ethical question: As trends emerge, how far are we willing to go in pursuit of greater certainty? For scientific validation, we might require greater certainty than an individual physician would require for clinical judgment—that is, for determining which treatment the patient should receive. Thus, the critical moral question is not informed consent, but the continuing risk-benefit analysis, especially as applied to present patient-subjects in relation to future patients. It is substantive rather than procedural: What degree of certainty for future patients is worth what risk to current patients?

COMPENSATION FOR INJURED RESEARCH SUBJECTS

Sometimes research subjects are injured despite all precautions. Injury is a risk of participation in research. Not all injuries can be foreseen, much less prevented. When subjects suffer research-related injuries, should they be compensated? A common assumption appears to be that, if a subject has been adequately informed about the risks of the research and consents to participate, all the possible injuries that are not the fault of the investigators should be accepted. Currently, subjects who suffer injuries in research can recover damages only under a notion of reparative justice, which requires a demonstration that there has been some fault, either negligence on the part of the investigators or failure to secure truly informed and voluntary consent. Institutions may act charitably toward such injured subjects, but in much research the injured party does not even receive free hospital coverage, much less disability coverage or payments to the family in case of death. Does society have an obligation to compensate injured research subjects even for no-fault injuries?

It is difficult to determine the number and seriousness of research-related injuries. According to a recent study, "the risks of participation in nontherapeutic research may be no greater than those of everyday life, and in therapeutic research, no greater than those of treatment in other settings."[28] Of the 93,000 subjects in nontherapeutic research covered by this study, 0.8 percent were reported injured: no one died, one subject was permanently disabled (although some doubt that the subject's stroke was caused by the research), 37 were temporarily disabled (reactions to drugs, corneal abrasions, electrical burns, and assault by another participant), and 673 suffered trivial injuries (discomfort, scars, colds, and mild allergic reactions). Of the 39,000 therapeutic-research subjects, 10.8 percent were reported injured; 43 deaths, 13 permanent disabilities, 937 temporary disabilities, and 3,253 trivial injuries were reported.

When such injuries occur, some people contend that society should act in a humanitarian way by providing compensation.[29] From this standpoint, we would be a better society—more humanitarian, kind, or benevolent—if we compensated research victims, but we would not be unjust if we did not. However, the injured research subject is not just another person who has "needs," but one who has taken risks for society's benefit through the advancement of medical knowledge.

Our society already recognizes an obligation to compensate persons who are injured in military service and, in some jurisdictions, Good Samaritans who are injured while aiding others, trying to prevent a crime, or assisting the police in apprehending suspected criminals (the last even being a legal duty in some places). Extrapolating from military service and Good Samaritan activities, we can identify at least three features that seem to give rise to an obligation on the part of society to compensate for injuries. These three features are clearly present in nontherapeutic research; I shall later consider whether they apply to therapeutic research. (1) The injured party accepts or is compelled to accept a position of risk ("positional risk").[30] Objective risks that the injured party would not otherwise have encountered emerge from the position accepted. (2) The activity is for the benefit of society, whatever any particular individual's motives may be. We can distinguish the general aim of the activity from the aims of any participant, whether researcher or subject. (3) Society, through the government or its agencies, conducts, sponsors, or mandates the practice in question. The third criterion provides some more or less official verdict that the activity is important for the society. We are interested in activities that involve positional risk for participants who objectively (if not subjectively) act on behalf and at the behest of society.[31]

When these features are present, the moral principle of fairness creates a societal obligation to participants, who can claim compensation at least for major injuries as their *right*. The obligation is voluntarily incurred by the society, through its support of the practice in question and its acceptance of the individual's participation. The obligation is based on the relationship between the parties in question and reflects the moral principle of fairness.

According to some defenders of compensation, subjects should be able to recover only for injuries not voluntarily assumed in consent to the research: *volenti non fit injuria* ("there is no injury to one who consents").[32] Because researchers cannot foresee all the injuries that might result from an experiment and cannot easily get subjects to understand and appreciate the risks, a subject's consent is rarely if ever fully informed. It is imperfect and incomplete and thus is not an assumption of all risks. Therefore, the society has an obligation to provide compensation for *some* injuries—those unforeseen and unanticipated.[33]

This viewpoint unfortunately perpetuates the notion that consent is the most important moral issue in experimentation. In fact, while it is a necessary condition for ethically justified research in normal circumstances, it is not, as we have seen, the only or even the first consideration. It authorizes the research to go forward with this individual. It does not, however, cancel society's moral obligation to provide compensation for subjects who assume a position of risk for the society's benefit under society's sponsorship or mandate. In military service, we do not discriminate between draftees and volunteers for purposes of compensating injuries. We do not say to the volunteer: "Look, you were well aware of what you were getting into. We cannot do anything for you."

Some contend that it is fair only to compensate participants

who have certain subjective motives. For them, a subject who
has calculated the risks and benefits of research to himself and
who has voluntarily assumed the risks should not be compensated for injuries. Such a subject has entered into a bargaining
situation, taken his chances, and lost. At most, society's obligation extends only to those who participate out of altruism, a
sense of duty toward the society, and the like. But it is really
impractical to try to determine the motives of participants.
Whatever their motives, subjects objectively assume positions
of risk in the name of and for the society. Their actions in
conjunction with society's actions such as mandating, sponsor-
ing, or conducting the research are sufficient to create the
obligation and correlative right.

To whom does society owe this obligation? The paradigm
case is the healthy volunteer who normally would not expect
to benefit medically from the procedure (although the volunteer may seek other benefits such as relief of boredom). The
research is nontherapeutic; it is designed to provide generaliz-
able knowledge. This paradigm case has the three features of
(1) positional risk (2) in a socially sponsored or mandated
practice (3) for social benefit.

But does society have an obligation to a sick or dying patient
who becomes a subject in therapeutic research designed to
generate knowledge but also to treat the patient? Consider the
randomized clinical trial, which mixes therapy and research
(e.g., the trials of simple and radical mastectomies, and of
coronary bypass surgery). The main features of nontherapeutic
research that give rise to a social obligation of compensation
persist in much therapeutic research: there is positional risk for
the benefit of society in socially sponsored or mandated research. The combination of roles of patient and subject with
the possibility of benefiting both oneself and others does not
cancel society's obligation.

The HEW Secretary's Task Force on the Compensation of
Injured Research Subjects (January 1977) held that society has
an obligation to compensate all persons who suffer injury as a

result of their participation in either therapeutic or non-therapeutic research provided that "injury" is construed narrowly:

> Harm, disability or death suffered by a subject at risk of biomedical and behavioral research . . . where such injury is (1) proximately caused by such research, and (2) on balance exceeds that reasonably associated with such illness from which the subject may be suffering, as well as with treatment usually associated with such illness at the time the subject began participation in the research.[34]

Obviously this standard requires complex judgments, and its application may be difficult in some cases. For example, if an experimental drug in a clinical trial extends a patient-subject's life by several years while causing deafness (which is not ordinarily associated with the disease or standard treatment), should compensation for deafness be offered? Or would the benefit of several additional years of life outweigh the loss of hearing so that on balance the injury would not be compensable?

Several other questions need to be answered before a feasible program of compensation can be developed. I have concentrated on one major reason for compensation: to discharge a moral obligation of compensatory justice required by the principle of fairness. Discharging this obligation could encourage volunteers for research and could allay some community and personal concerns about research. These gains provide additional reasons for doing what society should recognize as an obligation.[35]

Chapter 4

ALLOCATING
HEALTH CARE
RESOURCES

ISSUES IN ALLOCATION

Students of biomedical ethics have traditionally concentrated on issues in the patient-physician relationship. In recent years, however, they have devoted increasing attention to issues of biomedical ethics in public policy. Public policies, defined as "whatever governments choose to do or not to do,"[1] typically involve regulation (e.g., prohibition and control of an activity) and the allocation and distribution of benefits (e.g., goods and services) and burdens (e.g., taxation). Issues in the allocation of resources for and within health care are among the most difficult from the standpoint of ethics. My task is to analyze some of these issues. Although I shall argue for particular positions at several points, my main intention is to provide a map of several major issues. I shall emphasize the *content* of public policies, not the *processes* by which they are formulated and implemented.[2] I shall also avoid some broad and important questions of social ethics regarding the structure of the health care system in the United States (e.g., whether the current mix of private and public is desirable). While some policies may imply changes in the structure of the health care system, I shall limit my attention and analysis to policies of the allocation of resources for and within health care.

Another preliminary comment about my approach is necessary. How should we do ethics in relation to public policy? On the one hand, we could proceed by developing a systematic theory of justice or rights that could provide a basis for priorities in the allocation of health care resources. *A Theory of Justice* by John Rawls could be a model.[3] On the other hand, we could proceed by examining existing practices, institutions, and policies to determine their underlying principles and values. Then we could use these principles and values to illuminate priorities in allocation. Perhaps we would discover a plurality of principles and values, differently weighted in different policies, and possibly even incoherently stated and inconsistently applied. This second way of doing ethics is close to Albert Jonsen's and Lewis Butler's vision of "public ethics."[4] It has the advantages of concreteness and immediate relevance to policy, but it lacks the critical distance of the first approach.

I do not want to overemphasize the differences between these two approaches, much less to suggest that they are mutually exclusive or exhaust the possibilities. But my approach in this chapter is closer to the second one, since I do not defend the principles and values that I invoke. Instead, I examine the way several principles and values, such as equality, liberty, effectiveness and efficiency in the promotion of health, can illuminate our choices in the allocation of health care resources.

Our society affirms many principles and values that may come into conflict when we try to formulate public policies. For instance, the effective and efficient promotion of health may come into conflict not only with the principle of liberty (which I shall discuss later in connection with preventive health care) but also with the ideals of providing medical care "to each according to his needs" and providing equal access to medical care.[5] Let me describe the latter conflict. Rick Carlson contends that five major variables influence health, and he ranks them according to their importance: (1) environment, (2) life-style, (3) society, (4) genetics, and (5) medical care.

Medical care is the lowest on this list of influences on health and he gives it approximately 6 percent weight.[6] If his position is sound, to concentrate resources on *medical* care is to misallocate them. One does not have to agree with the "therapeutic nihilists," such as Ivan Illich, that medical care is pernicious (e.g., because it creates an attitude of dependence that leads individuals to abdicate their responsibility for their own health or because there is an increase in iatrogenic diseases) in order to concede that medical care is relatively ineffective in the promotion of health.[7] While medical care may have other values, such as reducing insecurity in crises of life, Paul Starr is right: "If one wishes to *equalize health, equalizing medical care* is probably not the most effective strategy."[8] But the promotion of health is not society's only goal. As long as medical care is perceived as important to health or at least increases our sense of security, perhaps we ought to promote *equal access* to it. Despite the apparent oddity of arguing for equal access to what is ineffective, the principle of equality may indicate that such a policy is morally defensible and even mandatory.

I want to concentrate on three major questions in the allocation of resources for and within health care:[9]

1. What resources (time, energy, money, etc.) should be put into health care and into other social goods such as education, defense, the elimination of poverty, and improvement of the environment?

2. Within the area of health care (once we have determined its budget), how much time, energy, money, etc., should we allocate for prevention and how much for rescue or crisis medicine?

3. Within either preventive care or rescue medicine, who should receive resources such as vaccines or artificial hearts when we cannot meet everyone's needs?

The first two questions involve "first-order determinations" or macroallocation decisions—how much of a good will be made available? The third question involves "second-order determinations" or microallocation decisions—who shall receive the available good?[10] I shall treat these questions as analytically distinct, but in practice they overlap and interact. Although second-order determinations presuppose first-order determinations, tensions and conflicts in the former may lead to a reassessment of the latter. Thus, tensions and conflicts in the allocation of scarce kidney dialysis and transplants in part led to the Federal Government's decision to allocate funds to cover practically everyone who needs dialysis or transplantation.

HEALTH CARE VS. OTHER SOCIAL GOODS

Current evidence does not indicate that our great expenditures in health and medical care in, say, the last twenty years have brought us closer to health. In particular, our exotic technologies offer only marginal returns in reducing morbidity and premature death. The advances in health in the last century can be accounted for largely by improvements in living conditions rather than in medical care. Therefore, the pursuit of some other social goods, such as improving the environment and reducing poverty, has beneficial effects on health.

If we accepted the World Health Organization's definition of health ("a state of complete physical, mental, and social well-being"), all social goods would relate directly or indirectly to health. Practically all allocation decisions would concern the aspects of health to be emphasized and the most effective and efficient means to their realization. But if we assume a narrower and more adequate definition of health (without developing the arguments for it at this point), we have to confront the conflict between health care, especially medical care, and some other social goods, not all of which serve as instruments to better health. For example, should hospitals always have priority over museums and opera houses? One philosopher, Antony Flew, has argued that "morally, so long as hospitals are needed, hospitals must always have priority over amusement parks" on the grounds that pain is not symmetrical with pleasure and that the prior or more fundamental duty is to alleviate pain.[11] But it is not evident (*a*) that hospitals are primarily to alleviate pain, and (*b*) that they should always take priority over all other social goods that do not contribute to the aim of hospitals, whether it is the alleviation of pain or some other goal. Health may be a condition for many values for individuals and the community, but it does not have finality or ultimacy. It is not true that when it comes to health, no amount is too much.

Paul Ramsey has said that he does not know how to go about resolving this first priority question—health care in relation to other social goods—because it is "almost, if not altogether incorrigible to moral reasoning" and "to rational determination."[12] Perhaps, as Ramsey suggests, it is basically a *political* question—one to be resolved through political processes that can reflect the values, preferences, and informal priorities of the society. Can one complain of *injustice* if a society puts more money into space programs or defense than health care? "Wrong" priorities may not be unjust unless there are certain basic needs or rights that must be satisfied for justice to be realized.

Suppose we say that just policies give to each according to their needs and that medical care is a basic human need. Medical needs are unpredictable, random, and overwhelming, according to one line of argument, and society ought to be prepared to meet those needs. Such an argument would depend on a vision of human life that we cannot assume in our society—a vision that would rank needs and make health the most important one. Even if we distinguish needs and wants, demands for health care appear to be virtually without limit. And we have to ask how much we are willing to devote to the provision of medical care which, as we have seen, may not be all that important for health.

Another line of argument is that there is what Charles Fried calls a right to a decent minimum of health/medical care,[13] and that society should make sure that there is enough in the budget to meet this need. An argument for equal access to medical care does not necessarily imply a minimum for individuals and thus for the health budget. It may only mean equal access to what is available. And what is available may be meager. But a right to a *decent minimum* establishes a base for individual medical care and, consequently, for the health budget. It would provide a standard for determining the minimum amount for the health care budget. But, again, in the absence of a shared vision of humanity, we may have to resort to the political process to define the decent minimum for individuals.

In short, to determine how to allocate resources for health care in relation to other social goods, we need to resolve several matters: the definition of health, its value, its causes, whether there is a right to a decent minimum of health/medical care, and what that minimum is.

PREVENTION VS. RESCUE OR CRISIS MEDICINE

Within the health care budget, how much should we allocate for *prevention* and how much for *rescue* or *crisis medicine?* This question is only one of several that could be raised and profitably discussed about allocative decisions within the health care budget. For example, another very important question concerns *basic research* vs. *applied research.* In response to Ivan Illich, who claims that modern medicine is a major threat to health, Dr. Lewis Thomas replies that we do not really have modern medicine yet.[14] Medicine has "hardly begun as a science." Most diseases cannot be prevented because we do not understand their mechanisms. Until we have more basic research, he contends, we will simply develop more and more "halfway technologies," such as transplanted and artificial organs, that merely compensate for the incapacitating effects of certain diseases whose course we can do little about. A halfway technology is designed to "make up for disease, or to postpone death." Usually it is very expensive and requires an expansion of hospital facilities. By contrast, a "high technology" based on an understanding of disease mechanisms is very simple and inexpensive. Compare the treatment of polio by halfway technologies, such as iron lung and support systems, with the simple and inexpensive high technology—the polio vaccine.

I want to concentrate on prevention and crisis or rescue medicine. Although this conflict rarely emerges in a clear and manageable form in debates about public policy, it is present and needs identification and analysis so that we can appreciate the "trade-offs" that we frequently, if unwittingly, make. *Prevention* includes strengthening individuals (e.g., through vaccines), changing the environment, and altering behavioral patterns and life-styles. As I have indicated, many recent commentators insist that the most effective and efficient way to improve the nation's health is through *prevention* since our current emphasis on rescue medicine now produces only marginal returns. DHEW's *Forward Plan for Health,* Fiscal Years 1977–81, holds: "Only by preventing disease from occurring, rather than treating it later, can we hope to achieve any major improvement in the Nation's health."[15]

This recommendation is at odds with our current macroallocation policies. For example, in 1976 expenditures for health amounted to 11.4 percent of the federal budget. When that amount (42.4 billion dollars) is assigned to four major determinants of health (human biology, life-style, environment, and the health care system), the results are striking: 91 percent went to the health care system, while 3 percent went to human biology, 1 percent to life-style, and 5 percent to environment.[16]

Nevertheless, the evidence for the effectiveness and efficiency of a preventive strategy to reduce morbidity and premature mortality by concentrating on human biology, life-style, and environment is by no means conclusive. The appropriate mix of preventive and rescue strategies will depend in part on the state of knowledge of causal links. Despite the dramatic example of polio, some other conditions, such as renal failure, are not the result of a single disease or factor. As a consequence, prevention appears to be only a remote possibility. In some cases prevention (which might involve extensive and expensive screening in order to identify a few persons at risk) may be less cost-effective than therapy after the disease has manifested itself. As Thomas suggests, our uncertainty in these areas is an argument for increased research.

Even if a preventive program (at least in certain areas) would be more effective and efficient, its implementation would not be free of moral, social, and political difficulties. Effectiveness and efficiency, or utility, are not the only relevant standards for evaluating policies of allocation of resources within health care (which is defined broadly and includes more than medical care). I shall concentrate on (1) the symbolic value of rescue efforts (what is symbolized about both the victim and the rescuer), (2) the duty of compensatory justice generated by the principle of fairness, (3) the principle of equal access, and (4) the principle of liberty.

1. Our society often favors rescue or crisis intervention over prevention because of our putative preference for known, identified lives over statistical lives. The phrase "statistical lives" (Thomas Schelling) refers to unknown persons in possible future peril.[17] They may be alive now, but we do not know which ones of them will be in future peril. Mining companies often are willing to spend vast sums of money to try to rescue trapped miners when they will spend little to develop ways to prevent such disasters even if they could save more lives *statistically* in the long run. At 240 million dollars a year, we could save the lives of 240 workers at coke ovens. We do not know which ones will be saved, and we are not likely as a society to respond enthusiastically to this expenditure. But we cannot ignore statistical lives in a complex, interdependent society, particularly from the standpoint of public policy.

The principle of equality is not violated by including statistical lives in public policy deliberations. It is not merely a matter of sacrificing present persons for future persons, for there are two different distinctions to consider: on the one hand, the distinction between *known* and *unknown* persons; on the other hand, the distinction between *present* and *future* peril.[18] Existing and known persons who may not be in present danger may be in future danger if certain preventive measures are not taken. Thus, preventive measures may aid existing persons who are at risk and not only future persons.

Following Max Weber, it is possible to distinguish between "goal-rational" *(zweckrational)* and "value-rational" *(wertrational)* conduct.[19] Conduct that is goal-rational involves instrumental rationality—reasoning about means in relation to ends. Conduct that is value-rational involves matters of value, virtue, character, and identity that are not easily reduced to ends, effects, or even rules of right conduct. There is thus an important distinction between *realizing* a goal and *expressing* a value, attitude, or virtue. In the context of debates about prevention and rescue intervention, the goal-rational approach concentrates on effectiveness and efficiency in statistical terms, while the value-rational approach focuses on the values, attitudes, and virtues that policies express.

This distinction between value-rational and goal-rational conduct may illuminate the 1972 congressional decision to make funds available for almost everyone who needs renal dialysis or transplantation. This decision followed widespread publicity in the media about particular individuals who were dying of renal failure. One patient was even dialyzed before the House Ways and Means Committee. Now we have a program that costs over a billion dollars each year. Some argue that this decision was an attempt to preserve society's cherished myth that it will not sacrifice individual lives in order to save money. Of course, we make those sacrifices all the time (e.g., when we fail to pass and enforce some safety measures). But society's myth is not as threatened when the sacrificed lives are statistical rather than identified. Hence, decisions to try to rescue identified individuals have symbolic value. It has been said that the Universalists believe that God is too good to damn human beings, and the Unitarians believe that human beings are too good to be damned. Similarly, the symbolic value argument suggests that rescue attempts show that individuals are "priceless" and that society is "too good" to let them die without great efforts to save them. This is society's myth. And, so the argument goes, when Congress acted to cover the costs of renal dialysis, it acted in part to preserve this myth, for the "specific individuals who would have died in the absence of the government program were known."[20] They were identified lives. The policy was value-rational, if not goal-rational.

Insofar as this argument focuses on the way rescue interventions symbolize the value of the victims, it encounters difficulties as a basis for allocative decisions. Consider two possibilities: (a) We keep the same total lifesaving budget but withdraw resources from *preventive* efforts in order to put them in *rescue* efforts so that we can gain the symbolic value of crisis interventions. As Charles Fried argues, "surely it is odd to symbolize our concern for human life by actually doing less than we might to save it," by saving fewer lives than we might in a maximizing strategy. (b) We keep the same prevention budget but take resources from other areas of the larger budget (cf. my discussion under "Health Care vs. Other Social Goods," above) so that we can increase crisis interventions. In this case, however, "we symbolize our concern for human life by spending more on human life than in fact it is worth."[21]

The symbolic-value argument focuses not only on the symbolic value of the victims but also on what is symbolized about the agents: the virtue and character of the society and its members, what is sometimes called "agent-morality." Conduct that is value-rational, in contrast to goal-rational, may thus be based on an answer to the questions Who are we? or Who shall we be? Allocation policies may be thought of as ways for the society to define and to express its sense of itself, its values, and its integrity. From this standpoint, it is possible to argue that rescue efforts should be important, if not dominant, in allocative decisions. As Lawrence Becker notes, "we have (rationally defensible) worries about the sort of moral character represented by people who propose to stand pat and let present victims die for the sake of future possibilities. One who can fail to respond to the call for help is not quite the same sort of character as one who can maximize prevention."[22] Although agent-morality has strong appeal, and no doubt influences many of our decisions, it is difficult to determine how much weight it should have in our policy deliberations.

2. In some situations the principle of fairness can generate a duty of *compensatory justice* that assigns priority to identified lives in present danger. In such situations society has an obligation to try to rescue individuals even though it departs from a strategy that would save more lives in the long run. These situations involve some unfairness because of an inequality in the distribution of risks which the society has assigned, encouraged, or tolerated. Suppose that a person who has worked in a coal mine under terrible conditions which should have been corrected is trapped in a cave-in or comes down with a disease related to his working conditions. Fairness requires greater expenditures and efforts for him in order to equalize his risks. Likewise, if society fails to correct certain environmental conditions that may interact with a genetic predisposition to cause some diseases, it may have a duty of compensatory justice. A policy of compensatory justice in health-related matters, of course, faces numerous practical difficulties, such as identifying causation. But it is important to underline the point that the principle of fairness can generate a duty of compensatory justice which sets limits on utility and efficiency in some situations. Those who argue that individuals voluntarily choose to bear risks and thus waive any claim to compensatory justice need to show that the individuals in question really understand the risks and voluntarily assume them (e.g., do the workers in an asbestos factory have an opportunity to find other employment, to relocate, etc.?). But even the voluntary assumption of risks should not always be construed as a waiver of a claim to compensatory justice when the person is injured (e.g., research-related injuries).[23]

3. If we include statistical lives in a preventive strategy, while allowing for compensatory justice, we still face difficult questions about *distributive justice,* particularly the principle of equality or equal access. It is not enough to maximize aggregate health benefits. Our policies should also meet the test of distributive justice, which is, indeed, presupposed by compensatory or corrective justice. For example, consider a program to reduce hypertension (high blood pressure) which affects approximately 24 million Americans and poses the risk of cardiovascular disease. In order to reduce the morbidity and mortality from cardiovascular disease, Milton Weinstein and William Stason propose an antihypertensive program on the basis of cost-effectiveness analysis. They recommend the intensive management of known hypertensives instead of public screening efforts. As they recognize, this proposal appears to be disadvantageous to the poor who would probably be unaware of their hypertensive condition because of their limited access to medical care. This inequity might be diminished by Weinstein's and Stason's proposal to give priority to target screening in black communities over community-wide screening, since hypertension is more common among blacks than among whites, and similarly to selective screening in low-income communities.[24]

The formal principle of equality, or justice, is "treat similar cases in a similar way." Of course, such a formulation does not indicate the relevant similarities. When we discuss equal access to medical care, we most often consider medical need, in contrast to geography, finances, etc., as the relevant similarity that justifies similar treatment. Suppose we decide that an effective and efficient strategy to improve the nation's health will not permit us to do all we could do in rescue or crisis medicine. A decision to forgo the development of some technology or therapy may condemn some patients to continued ill health and perhaps to death. Can such a policy be justified?

One possible approach that still respects the formal principle of justice and rules out arbitrary distinctions between patients (e.g., geography and finances) would exclude "entire classes of cases from a priority list." According to Gene Outka, it is more "just to discriminate by virtue of categories of illness, for example, rather than between rich ill and poor ill."[25] Society could decide not to allocate much of its budget for treatment of certain diseases that are rare and noncommunicable, involve high costs, and have little prospect for rehabilitation. The relevant similarity under conditions of scarcity would not be medical need but category of illness. While certain forms of treatment would not be developed and distributed for some categories of illness, care would, nonetheless, be provided. Patients would not be abandoned.

In the allocation of funds for research into the prevention and treatment of certain diseases, it is important to consider such criteria as the pain and suffering various diseases involve, their costs, and the ages in life when they are likely to occur.[26] By applying criteria such as pain and suffering, we might decide to concentrate less on killer diseases, such as forms of cancer, and more on disabling diseases, such as arthritis. Thus, says Franz Ingelfinger, national health expenditures would reflect the same values that individuals express: "It is more important to live a certain way than to die a certain way."[27]

One danger in establishing priorities among diseases should be noted: a decision about which diseases to treat may in fact conceal a decision about which population groups to treat since some diseases may be more common among some groups.[28] Injustice may result from these priorities.

4. The principle of *liberty* also poses some moral, social, and political difficulties for an effective and efficient preventive strategy. Mounting evidence indicates that a key determinant of an individual's health is his or her *life-style.* Leon Kass argues that health care is the individual's duty and responsibility, not a right.[29] And Lester Breslow offers seven rules for good health that are shockingly similar to what our mothers always told us! The rules, based on epidemiological evidence, are: don't smoke, get seven hours' sleep each night, eat breakfast,

keep your weight down, drink moderately, exercise daily, and don't eat between meals. At age forty-five, one who has lived by six of these rules has a life expectancy eleven years longer than someone who has followed fewer than four.[30] In his book *Who Shall Live?* Victor Fuchs contrasts the states of Utah and Nevada, which have roughly the same levels of income and medical care, but are at the opposite ends of the spectrum of health. For example, mortality for persons ages twenty to fifty-nine is approximately 39 percent higher in Nevada than in Utah. Fuchs asks:

> What, then, explains these huge differences in death rates? The answer almost surely lies in the *different lifestyles* of the residents of the two states. Utah is inhabited primarily by Mormons, whose influence is strong throughout the state. Devout Mormons do not use tobacco or alcohol and in general lead stable, quiet lives. Nevada, on the other hand, is a state with high rates of cigarette and alcohol consumption and very high indexes of marital and geographical instability. The contrast with Utah in these respects is extraordinary.[31]

On the one hand, we have increasing evidence that individual behavioral patterns and life-styles contribute to ill health and premature mortality. On the other hand, we have the liberal tradition that views life-styles as matters of private choice, not to be interfered with except under certain conditions (e.g., harm to others).

Each person has what Charles Fried calls a *life plan* consisting of aims, ends, values, etc. That life plan also includes a *risk budget,* for we are willing to run certain risks to our health and survival in order to realize some ends.[32] We do not sacrifice all our other ends merely to survive or be healthy. Our willingness to run the risk of death and ill health for success, friendship, and religious convictions discloses the value of those ends for us and gives our lives their style. Within our moral, social, and political tradition, the principle of liberty sets a presumption against governmental interference in matters of life-style and voluntary risk-taking. But that presumption may be over-ridden under some conditions. Let me make a few points about those conditions, which are similar to just war criteria:

a. An important goal is required to override liberty. One such goal might be *paternalism:* to protect a person even when his or her actions do not harm anyone else. This goal is rarely a sufficient justification for interference with liberty. Usually we require that restrictions of liberty be based, at least in part, on the threat of harm to others or to the society (e.g., compulsory vaccinations). We have difficulties with purely paternalistic arguments in requiring seat belts, helmets, etc. Another goal might be to *protect the financial resources of the community.* If we get national health insurance, we can expect increased pressure to interfere with individual liberty. Why? People simply will not want to have their premiums or taxes increased to pay for the *avoidable afflictions* of others. They will charge that such burdens are unfair.

b. To override the presumption against interfering with liberty, we need strong evidence that the behavior or life-style in question really contributes to ill health. This second standard must be underlined because there is a tendency to use a term like "health," which has the ring of objectivity, to impose other values without articulating and defending those values. In Albert Camus's novel *The Plague,* a doctor and a priest fighting the plague in an Algerian city engage in the following conversation. The priest says to the doctor: "I see that you too are working for the salvation of mankind." "That is not quite correct," the doctor replies. "Salvation is too big a word for me. I am working first of all for man's health." The danger is that "salvation" or "morality" or a certain style of life will be enforced in the name of health although it has little to do with health and more to do with the legislation of morality.

c. Another condition for overriding the presumption against interfering with liberty is that the interference be the *last resort.* Other measures short of interference, such as changing the environment, should be pursued and sometimes continued even when they are less effective and more costly than measures that restrict liberty.

d. A fourth condition is a reasonable assurance that the restriction will have the desired result as well as a net balance of good over evil.

e. Even when we override the principle of liberty, it still has an impact. It requires that we use the least coercive means to reduce risk-taking. For example, information, advice, education, deception, incentives, manipulation, behavior modification, and coercion do not equally infringe liberty. In addition to choosing the least restrictive and the least coercive means, we should evaluate the means on other moral grounds.

These considerations and others come into play when we try to determine whether, and which, incursions into personal liberty are justified. To allocate resources to prevention rather than to rescue is not a simple matter, for successful prevention may infringe autonomy and other moral principles.

COMPETITION FOR SCARCE MEDICAL RESOURCES

In either prevention or rescue, who should receive resources such as vaccines or artificial hearts when we cannot meet everyone's needs? While the first two questions covered issues of macroallocation, this third question focuses on microallocation decisions that hospitals and physicians have to make. It has been raised most dramatically for our generation by the allocation of kidney dialysis in the 1960s and early 1970s. (In dialysis, the functions of the kidneys are taken over by a machine that filters waste products such as urea from the patient's blood.) Access to scarce "kidney machines" was a matter of life and death for many people, and fortunate recipients were selected from the pool of medically acceptable candidates (i.e., those who would probably benefit from the dialysis) by the use of criteria of social worth or by some impersonal procedure such as queuing, lottery, or randomization. As I have already suggested, social discomfort with these microallocation decisions was one reason that federal legislation provided almost universal funding for kidney dialysis. No longer a scarce resource, dialysis is now provided to some patients even though it is not in their best interests.

Microallocation decisions are not new. Ancient Stoics, Jews, and Christians all discussed how to distribute scarce lifesaving resources among different individuals. For example, there was debate about what ought to be done when two survivors of a shipwreck simultaneously reach a floating plank that can support only one of them. Some Stoics held that "one should give place to the other, but that other must be the one whose life is more valuable either for his own sake or for that of his country." If these considerations are of equal weight, "one will give place to the other, as if the point were decided by lot or at a game of odd and even."[33] In general, Christians tended to emphasize self-sacrifice out of love in such situations. According to Ambrose, "Some ask whether a wise man ought in case of a shipwreck to take away a plank from an ignorant sailor? Although it seems better for the common good that a wise man rather than a fool should escape from shipwreck, yet I do not think that a Christian, a just and a wise man, ought to save his own life by the death of another, just as when he meets with an armed robber he cannot return his blows, lest in defending his life he should stain his love toward his neighbor."[34] Ambrose did, however, recognize the legitimacy of using force to defend innocent third parties. Several rabbis debated what should be done when two men who are on a journey through a desert have only one pitcher of water, enough to sustain one man but not both. One line of interpretation held that both should drink and die, but Rabbi Akiba held that "your life takes precedence over his life." The Jewish tradition tends to give greater weight to self-preservation than some strands of the Christian tradition. Some Jewish texts also recognize *utilitas* ("utility") but only when a person is choosing between two other human beings.[35]

Physicians can find little guidance for rationing in their tradition of medical ethics. According to the Hippocratic tradition, they are to benefit their patients; they are not advised on what to do when they cannot benefit all their patients who have equal needs. Thus, they have to look elsewhere for guidance. The closest analogies are in legal decisions in cases of killing survivors of shipwrecks to eat their flesh or jettisoning fellow passengers in order to save some lives when not all can survive.[36] Analogical reasoning is required because of the formal principle of justice: treat similar cases in a similar way. There are, of course, important dissimilarities between microallocation in health care and these legal cases: those involved in shipwrecks decide for themselves as well as for others, and often they kill rather than merely let die. But, as Paul Ramsey insists, there is no difference between these cases as far as the selection process is concerned.[37]

Microallocation is by no means exotic. It is often required for new techniques and drugs such as anesthesia, insulin, penicillin, and polio vaccine (in England) in addition to kidney dialysis. It also emerges in the neonatal intensive care nursery, and it will have to be faced when the totally implantable artificial heart becomes available.

There is general agreement about at least one standard of selection. Priority should be given to persons who can and probably will benefit from the procedure. It would be irrational and irresponsible not to consider medical acceptability. At the very least, it is a standard for determining the pool of candidates from which the final selection can be made. Whether it should also be used in the final selection is more controversial.

What factors should be included in judgments of *medical acceptability?* Answers will vary according to the medical problem and treatment. For example, various psychiatric factors, including "cooperativeness," were important for dialysis but less important for kidney transplantation. The dialysis patient is subjected to extreme pressures in part because of his dependence on the machine so many hours each week. Thus, it is not surprising that the incidence of suicide among patients on dialysis is "more than 100 times that of the general population."[38]

Medical-psychiatric criteria should not illicitly incorporate judgments of social worth and value. One way to purify medical-psychiatric criteria is to determine and apply them as though the resource is unlimited. By making scarcity irrelevant in judgments of medical acceptability, physicians would exclude only those who could not possibly benefit from the treatment.[39]

If the pool of medically acceptable candidates is too large, how should the final selection be made? Three major approaches, each expressing distinct constellations of values, compete for dominance. The first is the *use of objective criteria,* such as age, sex, and number of children in the family. But unless these criteria are simply arbitrary and perhaps discriminatory against certain classes such as old people, females, and single people, they have to be justified. And their justification will probably be either (*a*) medical-psychiatric (e.g., "children under age sixteen will have too many problems adjusting to this treatment") or (*b*) social (e.g., "we should give her priority because she has two children"). For example, age may be an arbitrary but objective standard, or it may reflect judgments of medical acceptability or social worth. If the justification is medical-psychiatric, what I have already argued is sufficient. If it is social, it is best considered in relation to utilitarian selection.

This second approach, *utilitarian selection,* assigns priority to persons who will probably contribute the most to society. It seeks the greatest good for the greatest number. Several arguments support utilitarian patterns of distribution in health care, but they are finally inadequate. Medical institutions and professionals are "trustees" for the social interest, and in rationing, "society 'invests' a scarce resource in one person as against another and is thus entitled to look to the probable prospective 'return' on its investment."[40] But, as I argued in the last two chapters, if society were to view the medical relationship merely as an instrument or tool for realizing broad societal values, it would destroy the relationship of "personal care." That relationship has its own integrity and value apart from its social productivity.[41]

In addition, it is important to distinguish levels of responsibility; not everyone should act in the same way or even in terms of the same standards. The physician is not a policy maker. His or her primary responsibility is to the patient, and society has good reasons for insisting on the primacy of this responsibility of personal care. Physicians should do all they can for their patients without counting society's resources and without taking into account the range of factors (e.g., statistical lives) that policy makers should consider. As Howard Hiatt contends, it is

> not fair to ask the physician or other medical-care pro-
> vider to set them [i.e. national priorities] in the context
> of his or her own medical practice. A physician or other
> provider must do all that is permitted on behalf of his
> patient. In that sense, the physician is or should be re-
> sponsible, with his patient and the patient's family, for
> setting priorities for that patient's management, within
> the limits available. The patient and the physician want
> no less, and society should settle for no less.[42]

The obligations of the physician and the bureaucrat are not identical. To whom and for what they are responsible depends, for example, on their positions and training and the moral principles that structure their roles. If we speak of medical personnel and institutions as trustees of society, we should not suppose that accountability requires making the physician's obligations identical with those of the policy maker.[43]

Another argument for utilitarian selection is that the third approach—queuing, chance, or randomization—is "literally irresponsible, a rejection of the burden." As Joseph Fletcher continues, "Its refusal to be rational is a deliberate dehumanization, reducing us to the level of *things* and blind chance." For Fletcher, the development of "criteria for selection" is "the number one task of medical ethics."[44] Likewise, Marc Basson contends that "random selection has no place in scarce medical resource allocation except when our primitive techniques for social value rating fail to distinguish among candidates in any way."[45] These proponents of utilitarian selection fail to see that rational people may have very good reasons for choosing impersonal mechanisms of allocation; these mechanisms may express and realize their principles and values better than any other method.

One major difficulty for utilitarian selection is the absence of clear and acceptable criteria of social worth in a pluralistic society. Because of the variety of criteria, different communities often make different judgments. For example, in the absence of clearly articulated standards, the anonymous lay committee that chose patients for dialysis in the Swedish Hospital in Seattle used such arbitrary standards as Scout leadership and church participation. Because rationing often reflects an unacknowledged scale of values, some defenders of utilitarian selection urge the use of attitude and opinion surveys in order to develop a scale of social values.[46] But even if utilitarian standards are articulated, defended, and fairly applied, a basic objection remains: we do not know enough to make total assessments of persons, particularly when such assessments determine life and death.

But the reasons for the third approach—*queuing, lottery, or randomization*—are not merely negative; they do not merely point to the inadequacies of utilitarian selection. (1) This third approach expresses some of our most important principles and values, particularly equality of opportunity and personal dignity, which cannot be reduced to one's social roles and functions. (2) Using a theological analogy, Paul Ramsey holds that in allocating scarce medical resources among equally needy persons, "an extension of God's indiscriminate care into human affairs requires random selection and forbids godlike judgments that one man is worth more than another."[47] (3) This third approach also supports trust between patients and health care professionals; such trust is difficult to maintain when patients are subjected to comparative assessments and are treated as means to some social end.[48]

These different systems of allocation often rest on different models of the cases that the system will handle. Should the system be designed for the "hard" or the "easy" cases? And which side should bear the burden of proof? How heavy should the burden be for those who would argue for exceptions? For example, according to societal values and defensible principles, it may be clear that a system should prefer the research scientist who is a person of high moral character and the father of five children over the convicted mass murderer. If this easy case is taken as the model, the system is likely to stress social worth and put the burden of proof on other approaches such as the use of chance when there are no substantial differences between the applicants. Although Nicholas Rescher includes social worth in his allocation system, he suggests that "if there are no really major disparities within this group . . . , then the final selection is made by *random* selection. . . ."[49]

If, on the other hand, hard cases are the model for the system, random choice, a lottery, or queuing ("first come, first treated") may be preferred. For example, if there is no "focused community," to use Ramsey's phrase, and if one must choose between physicians, lawyers, teachers, laborers, businessmen, etc.—each of whom is apparently dispensable from a functional standpoint and is roughly comparable in past contributions and moral virtue—how can one choose? By what criteria? By what certitude of society's needs and this candidate's indispensability? If these unfocused settings and hard cases are taken as normal, social worth judgments seem inappropriate and even impossible.

A pluralistic community may well become focused as a result of a disaster. In a focused community judgments about social worth are limited to the specific qualities and skills that are essential for the survival of that community; they are not total and do not concern the person as a whole. Ramsey gives three examples:[50] (1) the decision to allocate penicillin to men "wounded in brothels" rather than those wounded in battle among U.S. Armed Forces in North Africa in 1943 on the grounds that the former could more easily be made fit for combat; (2) the preservation of as many of the crew as are necessary for handling a lifeboat after a shipwreck; (3) triage in disaster medicine.

Triage functions in at least two different ways. First, it may sort out victims according to their medical needs: for example, those whose survival depends on immediate attention; those whose needs are not urgent; and those who will probably die regardless of treatment. Such classifications establish priorities of treatment—for example, in an emergency room after a major accident or on a battlefield. So far no considerations of social worth are involved. But triage may also compare patients in terms of their social worth in a focused community. For example, health care professionals with minor injuries may be treated first so they can help others. They are analogous to sailors on a lifeboat; some sailors should be given priority in order to save the others. But, as Ramsey notes, in a focused community, judgments about social worth are specific rather than general; they concentrate on the specific contributions to the community's survival, a precondition for other goods.[51]

Triage thus suggests a way to legitimate exceptions within an allocation system that uses chance. For example, a system could impose the following burden of proof on those who advocate an exception for patient X: only if X's contribution is indispensable to attaining (or preventing) a certain state of affairs, and only if society values (or fears) that result so much that it would deny Y a second transplant or would remove Z from treatment in order to save X.[52]

Rarely would this burden be met, in part because we are deeply committed to continuing to treat patients who are already in our care. To the best of my knowledge, no institution that used utilitarian selection was willing to reconsider the pool

of patients every few months to see if some new candidates
were more valuable than those already receiving dialysis. But
in a real emergency, or state of necessity, we might have to
pursue the lesser of two evils. That borderline case *(Grenzfall)*
may never arise. Although individuals are unique, they are
rarely indispensable in their social roles and functions. If an
emergency arises, we should treat it as a tragic exception to a
system of chance that best expresses and realizes our principles
and values.[53]

Chapter 5

THE ART
OF
TECHNOLOGY ASSESSMENT

TECHNOLOGY, ASSESSMENT, AND CONTROL

"It was the best of times, it was the worst of times, it was the age of wisdom, it was the age of foolishness." These words, which Charles Dickens uses for the French Revolution in *A Tale of Two Cities,* could easily apply to our discourse about technology. Positive and negative superlatives abound. We are quick to applaud or to disapprove. Rarely do we grasp the ambiguity of technology and the necessity of subtle and nuanced evaluations. Our public policies will not be responsible until we grasp this ambiguity and deal with it in relation to moral principles and values.

In the late 1950s and early 1960s, many commentators declared that the modern world had lost interest in, or the capacity to answer, big questions such as the meaning of life and the goals of our institutions. Social scientists such as Daniel Bell announced the "end of ideology," philosophers such as Peter Laslett observed that "political philosophy is dead," and theologians such as Harvey Cox noted the decline of religion. According to Cox, the secular city was emerging, and its inhabitants would be pragmatic and profane, interested only in what will work in this world. All these interpretations converged: individuals and communities are no longer interested in, or able to deal with, ideology, metaphysics, and mystery.[1] Some interpreters even went so far as to say that the important issues are merely technical and can be handled by the technicians or experts. President Kennedy expressed this viewpoint in the early '60s, when he held that the real issue today is the management of industrial society—a problem of ways and means, not of ideology. As he put it, "the fact of the matter is that most of the problems, or at least many of them, that we now face are technical problems, are administrative problems [requiring] . . . very sophisticated judgments which do not lend themselves to the great sort of 'passionate movements' which have stirred this country so often in the past."[2]

The obituaries for ideology, social and political philosophy, and religion were premature—as the events of the last twenty years have demonstrated. In the rapid growth of various religious communities and in the conflicts over civil rights, the war in Vietnam, abortion, and technology, it became clear that interest in the big questions was only dormant or overlooked in the rush to embrace new trends.

For the most part, those who wrote the obituaries for meaning and value in the modern world were quite sanguine about technological society and the technocrats who would run it without worrying about larger perspectives. But while they praised technological man, others such as Jacques Ellul viewed him with distrust and disdain.[3] However, their debates lacked subtlety and discrimination largely because the protechnologists and the antitechnologists tended to agree that the issue was technology as such (or at least modern technology as such). As a result, they obscured the importance of assessing and controlling particular technologies.

Unfortunately, these global perspectives endure. Two examples can be found in recent books. In *The Republic of Technology: Reflections on Our Future Community,* Daniel Boorstin, the Librarian of Congress, connects the growth of technology with the (alleged) decline of ideology: "Technology dilutes and dissolves ideology. . . . More than any other modern people we have been free of the curse of ideology."[4] Holding that we are most human when we are making and using tools, Boorstin is enthusiastic about technology as such.

An example of a global perspective that is negative toward technology (at least within one area of medicine) is Stanley Reiser's *Medicine and the Reign of Technology.* Reiser, a historian of medicine, traces the development of various diagnostic technologies such as the stethoscope and concludes that they have increasingly alienated physicians from patients. Because they provide external, objective signs, the physician no longer relies on his own personal contact with the patient for diagnosis. Thus, the physician concentrates on the measurable aspects of illness rather than on human factors. "Accuracy, efficiency, and security are purchased at a high price," Reiser contends, "when that price is impersonal medical care and undermining the physician's belief in his own medical powers." The physician, he says, must rebel against this "reign of technology."[5]

It is interesting that both Boorstin and Reiser choose "political" metaphors and images when they discuss technology: "republic," "reign," and "rebellion." And despite their different responses to technology, both appear to hold a form of technological determinism, either hard or soft. Technology determines social relationships, for example, between patient and physician. Not only are there problems with this determinism which makes technology an independent variable, but it is not accurate or helpful to approach technology as such, to offer global praise or blame. More precise and discriminate judgments are required if we are to reap the benefits and avoid the evils of particular technologies. One attempt in the last fifteen years to provide a way to control technologies through public policy is *technology assessment.* I want to examine the art of technology assessment, its possibilities and its limitations.

For our purposes, "technology" can be defined as the "systematic application of scientific knowledge and technical skills for the control of matter, energy, etc., for practical purposes."[6]

I shall concentrate on biomedical technologies: the technologies (techniques, drugs, equipment, and procedures) used by professionals in delivering medical care. Examples include insulin, the totally implantable artificial heart, kidney dialysis, CAT scanners, and in vitro fertilization.

We assess technologies in order to be able to "control" them responsibly through our public policies.[7] Public policy is a purposive course or pattern of action or inaction by government officials. Public policies designed to "control" technologies may operate in many different ways. The most typical and common controls are the allocation of funds (e.g., the decision to give research on cancer priority) and regulation or prohibition (e.g., the prohibition of the use of Laetrile). But it is also possible to permit and even to fund a technology while trying to control its side effects through other measures.

Control cannot be properly directed without an assessment of technology. The phrase "technology assessment" was apparently first used in 1966 by Philip Yeager, counsel for the House Committee on Science and Astronautics, in a report by the House Subcommittee on Science, Research and Development chaired by Congressman Emilio Q. Dadderio (D-Conn.), later the first head of the Office of Technology Assessment. Basically, technology assessment is a comprehensive approach, considering all the possible or probable consequences, intended and unintended effects, of a technology on society. It is thus multidisciplinary and interdisciplinary.

Against some interpreters and practitioners of technology assessment, I would argue that it is "an art form," not a science.[8] As an art form, it is basically the work of imagination which is indispensable for judgment-making. All sorts of methods can be used, and technology assessment should not be identified with any particular methods. Before policy makers had access to systems analysts, and the like, they consulted astrologers, and, on the whole, Hannah Arendt once suggested, it would be better if they still consulted astrologers! I want to show that technology assessment can be more than a narrow technique and that, as a broad approach, drawing on several different methods, it is an indispensable art.

THEOLOGICAL CONVICTIONS

Technology assessments will draw on theological (or quasi-theological) convictions as well as on moral principles and values. Before turning to the latter, I want to indicate how general theological convictions provide perspectives on and engender attitudes toward technology, often through perspectives on and attitudes toward nature.[9] It should be noted that Christian (and Jewish) convictions reflect certain tensions which may be creative or destructive.

On the one hand, the Christian tradition affirms the goodness of creation, holding that nature is not an enemy to be assaulted. On the other hand, it also leads to what Max Weber called "the disenchantment of the world" or "the rationalization of the world."[10] Its stress on God's transcendence tends to exclude spirits in nature who need to be approached with awe, and it thus frees nature for man's dominion.

Another tension can be seen in the distinction between sovereignty over nature and stewardship of nature. Although the Christian tradition has sometimes engendered (or at least supported) attitudes of human sovereignty over nature,[11] its dominant theme is human stewardship, deputyship, or trusteeship. While the sovereign is not accountable, the trustee is accountable to God and for what happens to nature. Human action takes place within a context in which humans are ultimately responsible to God as the sovereign Lord of life, Creator, Preserver, and Redeemer. Within this perspective of trusteeship, we cannot be satisfied with a short-term view of responsibility. For example, there is penultimate responsibility to and for future generations; it is not legitimate to slight this responsibility by asking, What has posterity ever done for us? And there is penultimate responsibility to and for nonhuman nature, not only because "nature bats last"!

Some theological critics reject the image of stewardship or trusteeship because it involves *dominium terrae.* But it is irresponsible to neglect or to repudiate human control over nature. The issue is not control (technology) but, rather, the ends, effects, and means of control (technology). This control is not total or unlimited; it is not absolute dominion. It is limited and constrained by nature itself, by moral principles and rules, and by ultimate loyalty and responsibility to God. It is not necessary or desirable to conceive these limits and constraints in terms of "rights" (e.g., rights of trees) as though we can imagine moral requirements only when we can invoke rights. However important rights are—and they are very important—we can conceive moral limits on our control of nature without appealing to them.

The ends of *dominium terrae* are also subject to criticism. If there is a hierarchy of interests, and if human interests are dominant, they should not be construed narrowly—for example, in terms of material goods. Nor should they exclude the goods of nature which are not reducible to human interests. Theologically, the propensity of human beings to construe their interests narrowly and to exclude nonhuman interests or goods is explained in terms of sin. Because humanity is fallen, its control over nature will frequently be misdirected and even destructive. In addition, as we will see when we discuss process later, procedures and mechanisms for reducing the effects of sin are indispensable; even though they cannot eradicate sin, they can lessen its destructiveness.

According to some theological critics, the image of stewardship or trusteeship is also suspect because it appears to separate human beings and nonhuman nature. To be sure, this image depends on a distinction between humanity and nature, but it does not imply an invidious separation. Humanity is part of nature. But, created in the image of God, it is a distinctive, even unique, part of nature. In addition, there may be a hierarchy of value with humanity at the apex. However much we need to emphasize the continuity between humanity and nature, discontinuity, at least as distinction, is still evident and important. Even as part of nature, humanity can still be a steward and trustee for nature.

Furthermore, to distinguish humanity and nature is not to deny their interdependence. Humanity should recognize its solidarity, its community of interests, with nature, because what affects nonhuman nature also affects humanity. It is not necessary or desirable, however, to focus on oneness or organic harmony or to develop a process theology in order to support an adequate ethic. It is possible, for example, to develop adequate limits on human control over nature from a perspective of conflict between humanity and nature in a fallen world. As Gerhard Liedke argues, such a perspective would hold that nonhuman nature is more than material, for, at the very least, it is a rival partner in a conflict. And it needs protection to ensure its participation as an equal in this conflict.[12] Furthermore, recognizing nature in this way is compatible with an attitude of awe and wonder that supports limits on human control over nature.

Although general theological (or quasi-theological) convictions provide perspectives and engender attitudes, they are not by themselves sufficient for the assessment of technologies. For such a task, we need an ethical bridgework or framework to connect these convictions, perspectives, and attitudes with judgments about technologies. Such a bridgework or framework will consist, in part, of general principles and values. But theological convictions, along with the perspectives they provide and the attitudes they engender, do not merely serve as warrants for moral principles and values. They also shape interpretations of situations to which we apply principles and values. Consider, for example, beliefs about death in debates about technologies to prolong and extend life. If a society views death as an enemy, always to be opposed, it will be inclined to provide funds to develop life-prolonging and life-extending technologies and to use them even when the expected quality of life is poor. An adequate critique would thus include convictions, perspectives, and attitudes that shape interpretations of situations, as well as moral principles and values.

Because it is not possible here to establish all the important connections between theological convictions, moral principles and values, and interpretations of situations, I shall assume several principles and values in order to trace their implications for the assessment of technologies.[13] Unless a single principle or value is accepted as overriding, conflicts and dilemmas are inevitable. As Guido Calabresi and Philip Bobbitt emphasize in *Tragic Choices,* tragedy is largely a cultural phenomenon: it depends on the principles and values of the individual or the society.[14] This point was underlined during a 1979 visit to the People's Republic of China with an interdisciplinary and inter-professional delegation interested in ethics, public policy, and health care. Frequently members of our delegation asked Chinese policy makers, health care professionals, and others how they handle some of our "problems" such as refusal of treatment. The most common response was: "That's not a problem here. It doesn't exist here." Sometimes this response reflected the stage of technological development; often, however, it reflected the unimportance of some Western principles and values such as autonomy, privacy (for which there is no Chinese word), and other ingredients of individualism.[15]

PRINCIPLES AND VALUES IN TECHNOLOGY ASSESSMENT

I now want to indicate how technology assessment might proceed and, in particular, what principles and values it ought to consider. Nothing in its logic requires that it be as narrow as it sometimes is. Its practitioners need not be what John Stuart Mill called "one-eyed men" attending only to the "business" side of life.[16]

1. Any technology assessment depends to a great extent on the principle of proportionality—proportion between the probable good and bad effects of technologies. This principle is expressed in various methods used to assess technologies, for example, cost-benefit analysis and risk-benefit analysis, which are only "new names for very old ways of thinking" (as William James said of pragmatism). They represent attempts to systematize, formalize, and frequently to quantify what we ordinarily do. For example, outside Canton, patients in a commune hospital formed their own risk-benefit analysis of traditional Chinese herbal medicine and Western medicine, both of which were available. They said, "Chinese medicine might not help you, but it won't hurt you; Western medicine might help you, but it also might hurt you."

I shall concentrate on *risk* and *benefit,* viewing risk as one sort of cost, i.e., cost as threat to safety, health, and life. The terms "risk" and "benefit" are perhaps not the best. Risk includes both amount or magnitude of harm and probability of harm. When we juxtapose benefit and risk, we are likewise interested in the magnitude and probability of benefit. It would be more accurate then to say that we need to balance the probability and magnitude of harm and the probability and magnitude of benefit. But since that expression is too cumbersome, I will use the common formulation of *risk-benefit analysis.*

Risk-benefit analysis involves what has been called "statistical morality."[17] Risks are everywhere, and one major question is how far we are willing to go in order to reduce the risks of premature mortality, morbidity, and trauma. Let us concentrate on mortality and ask the troubling question: How much is it worth to save a life (really to postpone death since lives are never really saved)? Or what is the value of a life? Consider the controversy over the Pinto. Apparently in 1973 Ford officials decided not to install a safety device that would prevent damage to the Pinto's gasoline tank in rear-end collisions. According to some reports, this device would have cost eleven dollars per vehicle or 137 million dollars for the whole production run. It is not accurate to say that Ford valued human life at eleven dollars. Rather, using a figure of approximately $200,000 per life, it concluded that the safety device should not be used because its costs outweighed its benefits.[18]

Economists propose two different ways to determine the value of life.[19] First, discounted future earnings. This approach tends to give priority to young adult white males. Thus a program to encourage motorcyclists to wear helmets would be selected over a cervical cancer program. Second, a willingness to pay. The question is not how much we would be willing to pay in order to avoid certain death, but how much we would be willing to pay to reduce the risk of death. How is willingness to pay determined? By finding out how much all those who are affected would be willing to pay, summing up the individual amounts, and then dividing by the anticipated number of deaths prevented. While it might be possible to study actual behavior (e.g., in the workplace), one promising approach uses opinion polls to determine, for example, how much a community would be willing to pay in taxes for a technology that would reduce the chances of death after a heart attack.

Although it may be impossible to avoid valuing lives (at least implicitly) in technology assessment, criticisms abound. Religious critics contend that life has infinite or absolute value. But their criticism is not serious insofar as it is directed against policies that do not do everything possible to reduce the risk of death. Judaism and Christianity, to take two examples, do not hold that life is an absolute value, superior to all other values. Both traditions honor martyrs who refuse to value life more highly than other goods such as obedience to the divine will. Furthermore, there is a difference between negative and positive duties, and the duty not to kill is more stringent than the duty to save lives.

Other critics hold that it is immoral to put a value on life. But we all have life plans and risk budgets.[20] Our life plans consist of aims, ends, and values, and our risk budgets indicate the risks to our health and survival we are willing to accept in order to realize some other goods. Health and survival are conditional, not final, values. A society might justly choose to put more of its budget into goods other than health and survival, as I argued in the previous chapter. Such a choice may be more political, i.e., to be resolved through the political process in terms of the community's values, or even aesthetic. One way to make this choice is to determine a community's willingness to pay for different goods.

An extension of these religious and moral objections opposes the calculation of consequences. Utilitarianism has sometimes been depicted as "ethics in cold blood." But, as I will argue later, consequences are always morally relevant even if they are not always morally decisive. This objection to calculation of consequences may simply be an objection to doing self-consciously and openly what we have to do. For example, Steven Rhoads argues that we should do a little dissembling since to put a public value on life would shock the community and perhaps lead to callousness.[21] In effect, he offers consequentialist grounds for not openly pursuing consequentialism.

These various objections to valuing lives do not hold. For the most part, they are not even aimed at the right targets. And it would be useful for us as individuals and members of a community to ask how much we are willing to spend to reduce the risk of death (in brief, to put a value on life).

It is obvious that value considerations determine what counts as benefit and what counts as harm. They also determine how much particular benefits and harms count, how much weight they should have in the calculation. An adequate risk-benefit analysis needs to keep in play a wide range of values to identify, weight, and balance benefits and harms. Analysts tend to prefer the hard, quantifiable variables, rather than the soft variables that are less susceptible to quantification. But a "narrow" cost- or risk-benefit analysis fails to convey the richness of our moral values and principles.

2. Value considerations not only shape our perceptions of

benefits and harms, they also "dictate the manner in which uncertainty as to the potential adverse consequences will be resolved."[22] To some analysts, the absence of evidence that harm will result is taken as evidence that the harm will not result, and so forth. The resolution of uncertainty, then, will reflect the value judgments of the analyst, whether he uses his own values or reflects the society's values. Description and evaluation cannot be separated even in the determination of the probability of harm because of "opposing dispositions or outlooks toward the future" such as confidence and hope or fear and anxiety.[23]

In the face of uncertainty, a procedural suggestion seems justified.[24] In the past, technology has been presumed innocent until proven guilty. ("Guilt" and "innocence" are used metaphorically to refer to risk-benefit analysis.) But in the light of our experiences in the last twenty years, we cannot be satisfied with this approach: we should, perhaps, presume that technology is guilty until proven innocent. The burden of proof and of going forward should be placed on the advocates of a technology who hold that its benefits will outweigh its harms. Such a shift in the *onus probandi* would not signal opposition to technological development. It would only indicate that we have not been sufficiently attentive to the harmful side effects and second-order consequences in technological development and that we intend to correct this deficiency.

A version of this procedure is mandated for the Food and Drug Administration, which cannot approve drugs for use outside research until they have been shown to be safe and efficacious. In effect, research may go forward (within the limits sketched in Chapter 3, "Human Subjects in Research"), research may even be funded (in accord with priorities sketched in Chapter 4, "Allocating Health Care Resources"), but let's not introduce a technology until we have determined with a reasonable degree of assurance that its probable benefits will outweigh its probable harms. This procedure will not harass or arrest technology.

3. It is not sufficient for a technology to have a favorable risk-benefit ratio; its proponents should also show that its risk-benefit ratio is more favorable than alternative technologies or even no technology at all. For example, if both X and Y have favorable risk-benefit ratios, they may not be equally acceptable if Y's ratio is more favorable. Many critics of technology call on society to consider alternative technologies, particularly technologies that emphasize the values of smallness and the integrity of person, community, and nature.[25] To a great extent, the issue is again the range of values that should be invoked for risk-benefit analysis.

4. We should seek to minimize risks even by *some* reduction in the probability and amount of the benefit we seek, if that is the only way to minimize the risks. Because we have duties to do no harm and to benefit others, we are responsible for balancing harms and benefits in an imperfect world. But, *ceteris paribus,* the principle of not harming others (including imposing risks) takes priority over the principle of benefiting others; thus, we should minimize risks even at some reduction in the magnitude and/or probability of the benefit. Although this principle is sound, it is difficult to specify how far we should go to minimize risks short of making it impossible to realize the benefit we seek.

5. In the long run, "the reversibility of an action should . . . be counted as a major benefit; its irreversibility a major cost."[26] Thus, reversibility of a technology and its effects should be preferred over irreversibility. Why should reversibility have this privileged position? Surely, if we could realize the ideal social order on earth, we would prefer that it be irreversible and imperishable. But precisely because of the *uncertainties* about probabilities and magnitudes of benefits and harms, we should be particularly cautious about technologies with apparently irreversible effects. The "preservation of future options" is an important goal, and it requires, for example, special concern of the destruction of an animal species and about nuclear waste.

Let me summarize these points about the principle of proportionality, the first consideration in technology assessment. We should balance the probabilities and amounts of benefits and harms. Value considerations will influence all aspects of the balance, including what counts as benefits and harms, how much they count, and how uncertainty is to be resolved. If lives are valued in public policy by determining how much people are willing to pay, the process of valuing lives is not inherently objectionable and may even be illuminating. Procedurally, the advocates of a technology should demonstrate its innocence before it is implemented and should show that its risk-benefit ratio is more favorable than any alternative technologies. We should minimize risks even when we reduce (within limits) the probability and amount of benefit. Finally, reversibility is a benefit, irreversibility a cost.

LIMITING PRINCIPLES

Many flaws in contemporary technology assessments can be traced to the perspective of utilitarianism—the moral, social, and political doctrine that acts and policies are to be judged by their consequences and effects. It is an end-result view of life. After my praise for the principle of proportionality, the reader may wonder whether I am not at least a "closet utilitarian." After all, isn't the principle of proportionality roughly what the utilitarians mean by the principle of utility—maximizing net benefit relative to harm? Any adequate moral, social, or political theory must include the principle of proportionality or the principle of utility. In a world that is not ideal, it is impossible always to do good and to avoid harm. Often doing good produces at least the risk of harm. The principle of proportionality or utility requires that we weigh and balance these benefits and harms when they come into conflict and that we try to produce a net benefit (or, when considering only bad states of affairs, the best of the alternatives). Whatever we call this principle, it is required by any adequate morality.

But we can accept the principle of proportionality or utility without accepting utilitarianism, which may be stated more sharply as the doctrine that right and wrong are determined *only* by the consequences of acts or policies. It makes the utility the *only* principle (act-utilitarianism) or the *primary* principle (rule-utilitarianism). And it distorts many technology assessments by restricting the range of relevant moral considerations. In particular, it concentrates on aggregative rather than distributive matters and it ignores other moral limits such as "rights" (which it frequently translates into "interests").

Utilitarian assessors sum up the interests of various individuals and groups to be affected by the technology, and they use this summation to determine our policy toward that technology. Although they may take account of wider and wider ranges of impacts and interests, they frequently overlook how burdens and harms are distributed. "Acceptable level of risk" of a technology, for example, should not be considered only in terms of the summed-up interests of the society. Principles of justice require that we consider the distribution of risks and benefits.

This issue can be sharpened by an examination of four possible patterns of distribution of risks and benefits. (1) The risks and benefits may fall on the same party. For example, in most therapy, the patient bears the major risks and stands to gain the major benefits. (2) One party may bear the risks, while another party gains the benefits. For example, in nontherapeutic research, the subject bears risks, while others in the future will gain the benefits. Or we may gain the benefits of some technologies that will adversely affect future generations. (3) Both parties may bear the risks, while only one party gains the benefits. For example, a nuclear-powered artificial heart would benefit the user but would impose risks on other parties as well as on the user. (4) Both parties may gain the benefits, while only one party bears the risks. For example, persons in the vicinity of a nuclear power plant may bear significantly greater risks than other persons who also benefit from the plant. These patterns suggest the importance of considerations of distributive justice. As an Advisory Committee on the Biological Effects of Ionizing Radiations reports:

> For medical radiation, as well as for certain uses of radiation in energy production, the problem of balancing benefits and costs is complicated by issues of ethics and discrimination. As an example, increased years of life expectation or increased economic productivity can be a useful measure of health benefit in some contexts. If, however, these parameters are used to balance the benefit-cost equation against the elderly with limited life expectancy or those with limited productivity, important values of society will have been overlooked.[27]

Utilitarianism in technology assessment often fails to take account of other limits because of its particular view of rationality. Max Weber drew classic distinctions between types of social action: "goal-rational" *(zweckrational),* "value-rational" *(wertrational),* affective, and traditional types of action. For our purposes, the first two, which I introduced in Chapter 4, are the most important. Value-rational conduct involves "a conscious belief in the absolute value of some ethical, aesthetic, religious, or other form of behaviour, entirely for its own sake and independently of any prospects of external success."[28] Goal-rational conduct involves reasoning about means to ends. It is a form of "instrumental rationality," involving the choice of effective (and efficient) means to given ends. It has been dominant not only in technology but also in technology assessment. By stressing limits, I have tried to include another type of rationality that may modify instrumental rationality by setting boundaries and constraints on the pursuit of goals.

Instrumental rationality tends to exclude value-rational considerations because they do not fit easily into the schema of means and ends. Just as I suggested about policies of the allocation of resources, we might choose policies toward technologies not because they *achieve* certain goals, but because they *express* certain values. They are expressive, symbolic, or representative. This range of considerations frequently involves *gestures,* not only *tasks.* For example, we might approach nature to make it serve our needs, or to express a certain attitude toward or relationship with it. As Laurence Tribe indicates, technology assessors typically ask what are society's current values regarding nature and they treat nonhuman life merely in relation to those values. But suppose society asked seriously, How should we value nature, including wildlife? And suppose the society came to the conclusion that it should treat nature with respect. Although this conclusion would not necessarily imply that the society would never give human interests priority over nature, "the very process of according nature a fraternal rather than an exploited role would shape the community's identity and at least arguably alter its moral character." As Tribe suggests, the decision maker's own identity might be at stake, for in choosing policies toward technologies, "the decision-maker chooses not merely how to achieve his ends but what they are to be and who he is to become."[29] Who are we and who shall we be? These are considerations of agent-morality that do and should influence our technology assessments.

PROCESS

One critical issue in technology assessment is often overlooked: process. Process is largely a matter of who should decide—that is, who should make the assessment, and how. It is possible to argue that technology assessors do not overlook process. Rather, they judge processes by their results. They ask whether particular processes "pay off" in producing the best possible outcomes—that is, the best possible predictions, evaluations, and controls of technology. When this judgment of processes by their results is combined with the view that we should judge technologies by their predicted consequences for human interests, as measured by preferences, there is one obvious conclusion: the *experts* should make the assessment. This

viewpoint simply perpetuates the myth of the end of ideology
even while trying to control technology.

Its critics are numerous and vocal. Many of them are concerned with processes of evaluation and decision-making in
some independence of their results. In technology assessment,
the demand for public participation has become widespread
and has encouraged the language of "participatory technology."[30] The World Council of Churches Church and Society
Conference on "Faith, Science and the Future" at the Massachusetts Institute of Technology in July 1979 emphasized "a
just, participatory and sustainable society." As the general secretary of the WCC, Philip Potter, put it in his address at the
MIT conference, "a just and sustainable society is impossible
without a society which is participatory." He continued:

> In the present situation of science and technology, they
> are not really participatory, or rather they are forced to
> be biased on the side of those who wield economic and
> political power. There is little sign that they are on the
> side of the oppressed, the deprived and the marginalized,
> or simply the people.[31]

It is no exaggeration to claim that "the central issue in technology assessment concerns democratic theory."[32] Involving the
public, and especially the individuals and groups affected by
the technology, expresses the value of equal concern and respect. It should be built not so much on anticipated results as
on the right to treatment as an equal.[33] Processes of public
participation in technology assessment are essential to embody
this right to treatment as an equal, as one whose wishes,
choices, and actions count. In addition, fairness, a principle
derived from the principle of equal concern and respect, applies to specific procedures that may be used for public participation (e.g., adversary hearings and public forums). These
values and principles are independent of the results of the
procedures and processes.

Emphasizing that technology requires a "new ethics of long-range responsibility," Hans Jonas notes the "insufficiency of representative government to meet the new demands on its normal principles and by its normal mechanics."[34] In a lighter vein, H. L. Mencken once said, "I do not believe in democracy, but I admit that it provides the only really amusing form of government ever endured by mankind." He went on to describe democracy as "government by orgy," an orgy of public opinion. Obviously, it is necessary to devise procedures and mechanisms that can both satisfy independent principles and values and sustain effective and disciplined public participation in technology assessment. The creation of such procedures and mechanisms may presuppose that we transcend interest-group liberalism.

TEMPORAL PERSPECTIVE

As currently practiced, technology assessment tends to "find opportunities for making judgments and taking action only at those points in which a new development in technology occurs."[35] Why? Perhaps because the utilitarianism back of much technology assessment is forward-looking, or because many assessors believe that what we now have is good, or because they believe that we cannot undo what has already been done. Whatever the reason, technology assessment for the most part predicts and evaluates for the future and is less interested in the evaluation of technologies already developed. Langdon Winner argues that we need not only "technology assessment" but also "technology criticism," which can look at the past and the present as well as the future, which can look at long-term trends of technological development as well as at particular technologies, and which can look at the society as well as at the technologies it produces.[36]

Winner's concerns are legitimate, but technology assessment, properly understood, can encompass them. It should be an ongoing process, dealing not only with the introduction of a technology but also with its impact as it is implemented. For example, there was no systematic assessment of the technology of renal dialysis in the 1950s and 1960s, but it has received careful scrutiny since its introduction, widespread use, and funding by the Government. While it is difficult to make adjustments once societal momentum has reached a certain point, we have learned and are continuing to learn from the experience with dialysis, and our experience may improve our policies in other areas. Among the numerous questions that remain about dialysis are whether it is worth the cost (already over one billion dollars a year), whether the money could have been spent better elsewhere, and whether we are able to cope with the successes of technologies (e.g., prolongation of life vs. quality of life of dialysis patients). Nevertheless, our struggle with these questions, and others, may illuminate present and future technology assessments.

Another point needs to be made about temporal orientation. Historical perspective may bring a cautionary tone to discussions of technology assessment. In a fine essay, entitled "Technology Assessment from the Stance of a Medieval Historian," Lynn White, Jr., directs our attention away from the easily measured factors to what he calls the "imponderables" and insists that technology assessment requires "cultural analysis" since the impact of a technology is filtered through the culture and the society.[37] Among his several case studies is alcohol, which was distilled from wine as a pharmaceutical at Salerno, the site of Europe's most famous medical school. How, he asks, could anyone have offered an assessment of alcohol in the twelfth century? Alcohol was praised in medieval literature as a pharmaceutical with beneficial effects for chronic headaches, stomach trouble, cancer, arthritis, sterility, falling or graying hair, and bad breath. It was supposed to be good for people who had a "cold temperament." But then widespread drunkenness and disorder became problems. To shorten the history, we have problems of traffic deaths and cirrhosis of the liver. White observes, "A study group eight centuries ago, equipped with entire foresight, would have failed at an assessment of alcohol as we today fail."

Although White's point is not always clear, it appears to be that technologies touch on many aspects of life (e.g., psychological and sociological factors) that cannot be determined with great precision. What will happen in the interactions between technologies and society, culture, and psyches is an "imponderable." His lesson is salutary. History is ironic, and we can only be modest about (*a*) our ability to *predict* effects, (*b*) our ability to *assess* effects, and (*c*) our ability to *control* effects. It is true, as a character in *Death Trap* puts it, that "nothing recedes like success." While modesty is in order because our abilities are indeed limited, we have no choice but to try to predict, to assess, and to control in the light of moral principles and values.[38]

NOTES

Introduction

1. See Miriam Siegler and Humphry Osmond, *Patienthood: The Art of Being a Responsible Patient* (Macmillan Publishing Co., 1979).

2. James F. Childress, "A Response to [Ronald Green] 'Conferred Rights and the Fetus,'" *Journal of Religious Ethics,* Spring 1974, pp. 77–83.

3. See Tom L. Beauchamp and James F. Childress, *Principles of Biomedical Ethics* (Oxford University Press, 1979).

4. See John Rawls, *A Theory of Justice* (Harvard University Press, 1971), pp. 40–45, 243–251, 339–342, *et passim.*

5. John Stuart Mill quoted Francis Bacon on *media axiomata* to indicate what he called "intermediate principles" (and, elsewhere, "subordinate principles") to use in applying the ultimate principle(s): "As mankind are much more nearly of one nature, than of one opinion about their own nature, they are more easily brought to agree in their intermediate principles, *vera illa et media axiomata,* as Bacon says, than in their first principles" (John Stuart Mill, "Bentham," in *Utilitarianism, On Liberty, Essay on Bentham,* ed. with an intro. by Mary Warnock [New American Library, Meridian Books, 1974], p. 119, cf. p. 276). The idea of "middle axioms" was used in ecumenical circles by J. H. Oldham and William Temple and developed by John C. Bennett in *Christian Ethics and Social Policy* (Charles Scribner's Sons, 1946), pp. 77ff. See the very helpful analysis in David H. Smith, *The Achievement of John C. Bennett* (Herder & Herder, 1970), pp. 140–156. Although it is often used in consequentialist theories, the idea of *media axiomata* may nevertheless be illuminating for a pluralist

theory. They are stronger than mere guidelines even though they may
lack broad generality and universality.

CHAPTER 1
PATERNALISM AND THE PATIENT'S RIGHT TO DECIDE

1. Robert W. Allen, "Informed Consent: A Medical Decision,"
Radiology, April 1976, pp. 233–234. This case appears in Beauchamp
and Childress, *Principles of Biomedical Ethics,* p. 255.

2. This case, based on a news report by Martha M. Hamilton in
The Washington Post, Nov. 14, 1974, was prepared by James J.
McCartney for Beauchamp and Childress, *Principles of Biomedical Eth-
ics,* pp. 260–261.

3. This case is based on material in Jay Katz, Joseph Goldstein, and
Alan M. Dershowitz, *Psychoanalysis, Psychiatry, and Law* (Free Press,
1967), pp. 552–554, 710–713. See also Robert A. Burt, *Taking Care
of Strangers: The Rule of Law in Doctor-Patient Relations* (Free Press,
1979), Ch. 2, where this case is discussed in detail.

4. This case is quoted from Sharon H. Imbus and Bruce E. Zawacki,
"Autonomy for Burn Patients When Survival Is Unprecedented,"
New England Journal of Medicine, Aug. 11, 1977, pp. 308–311.

5. This description of Talcott Parsons' position is drawn entirely
from one of his recent statements, "The Sick Role and the Role of the
Physician Reconsidered," *Millbank Memorial Fund Quarterly,* Summer
1975, pp. 257–278. See also Talcott Parsons, *The Social System* (Free
Press, 1951), pp. 428–479, and "Definitions of Health and Illness in
the Light of American Values and Social Structure," in E. Gartley Jaco
(ed.), *Patients, Physicians and Illness* (Free Press of Glencoe, 1958).
Parsons' most recent discussion of these themes does not deny paternalism and inequality but it also stresses a "collegial association"; see
Parsons, "Epilogue," in Eugene B. Gallagher (ed.), *The Doctor-Patient
Relationship in the Changing Health Scene,* publication of Geographic
Health Studies, John E. Fogarty International Center for Advanced
Study in the Health Sciences, DHEW Publication No. (NIH) 78-
183 (Washington, D.C.: U.S. Government Printing Office, 1978),
pp. 445–455.

6. Robert Nozick, *Anarchy, State, and Utopia* (Basic Books, 1974).

7. Ronald Dworkin, *Taking Rights Seriously* (Harvard University
Press, 1977), esp. Chs. 11 and 12. See also Ronald Dworkin, "Liberalism," in Stuart Hampshire (ed.), *Public and Private Morality* (Cambridge University Press, 1978).

8. For this distinction between strong and weak paternalism, see

Joel Feinberg, *Social Philosophy* (Prentice-Hall, 1973), pp. 50–51. Other important discussions of paternalism include Gerald Dworkin, "Paternalism," in Richard A. Wasserstrom (ed.), *Morality and the Law* (Wadsworth Publishing Co., 1971), pp. 107–126; Jeffrie G. Murphy, "Incompetence and Paternalism," *Archiv für Rechts-und-Sozialphiloso-phie* 60 (1974), pp. 465–486; John D. Hodson, "The Principle of Paternalism," *American Philosophical Quarterly,* January 1977, pp. 61–69; Tom L. Beauchamp, "Paternalism and Biobehavioral Control," *The Monist,* January 1977, pp. 62–80; Glenn C. Graber, "On Paternalism and Health Care," in John W. Davis, Barry Hoffmaster, and Sarah Shorten (eds.), *Contemporary Issues in Biomedical Ethics* (Humana Press, 1978), pp. 233–244; and Bernard Gert and Charles M. Culver, "The Justification of Paternalism," *Ethics,* January 1979, pp. 199–210.

9. See *Application of the President and Directors of Georgetown College,* 331 F. 2d 1000 (D.C. Cir.), certiorari denied, 377 U.S. 978 (1964). Excerpts appear in Beauchamp and Childress, *Principles of Biomedical Ethics,* pp. 261–262.

10. Rawls, *A Theory of Justice,* p. 249.

11. See note 4, above.

12. *Medical World News,* Jan. 22, 1979, p. 37. For the proceedings of the NIH (National Institutes of Health) Consensus Development Conference in Supportive Therapy in Burn Care, see *Journal of Trauma,* November 1979, Supplement, esp. pp. 876–877.

13. *Medical World News,* Jan. 22, 1979, p. 39.

14. See Case No. 228, "A Demand to Die," *Hastings Center Report,* June 1975, p. 9. See also Burt, *Taking Care of Strangers,* Ch. 1, for a thorough discussion of this case.

15. Wendy Carlton, *In Our Professional Opinion . . . : The Primacy of Clinical Judgment Over Moral Choice* (University of Notre Dame Press, 1978), pp. 5–6.

16. Although the ethos and practices should promote rather than merely preserve autonomy, I have emphasized the latter—autonomy as a side-constraint rather than as a goal.

17. For a fuller statement of these tendencies, see Carlton, *In Our Professional Opinion . . . ,* pp. 6–8, 178–179, *passim.*

18. This chapter is reprinted in revised form with permission from Virginia Abernethy (ed.), *Frontiers in Medical Ethics: Applications in a Medical Setting,* Copyright 1980, Ballinger Publishing Company. It was presented as a lecture in a symposium honoring Harry S. Abram at Vanderbilt University School of Medicine (1979), as one of the 1980 Willson Lectures at Earlham School of Religion, as one of the 1980 Wickenden Lectures at Miami University (Ohio), and at the

College of Physicians and Surgeons of Columbia University (while I was a visiting professor in the Department of Rehabilitation Medicine), Berea College, Bethany College, and the School of Medicine of the University of Chicago. An earlier version was presented at Washington and Lee University and appeared in Louis W. Hodges (ed.), *Social Responsibility: Journalism, Law, Medicine,* Vol. IV (Washington & Lee University, 1978). I am grateful to these institutions and to friendly critics of my lectures, particularly John Downey, whose perspectives have been very helpful.

CHAPTER 2
TO LIVE OR LET DIE

1. Edward Bond, *Bingo: Scenes of Money and Death* (London: Eyre Methuen, 1974), p. 42.

2. See Paul Ramsey and Richard A. McCormick, S.J. (eds.), *Doing Evil to Achieve Good: Moral Choice in Conflict Situations* (Loyola University Press, 1978).

3. James Rachels, "Active and Passive Euthanasia," *New England Journal of Medicine,* Jan. 9, 1975, pp. 78–80. For a fuller discussion, see Beauchamp and Childress, *Principles of Biomedical Ethics,* Ch. 4, and Bonnie Steinbock (ed.), *Killing and Letting Die* (Prentice-Hall, 1980).

4. Gilbert Meilaender, "The Distinction Between Killing and Allowing to Die," *Theological Studies,* September 1976, pp. 467–470. While there are important similarities between Meilaender's and Paul Ramsey's positions, Ramsey emphasizes the historical influence of Christianity without indicating clearly whether he views certain religious perspectives as logical presuppositions of the distinction between killing and letting die. See Paul Ramsey, *Ethics at the Edges of Life: Medical and Legal Intersections* (Yale University Press, 1978). In their profound discussion of the theological convictions that require the moral prohibition of euthanasia and suicide and yet authorize letting die in some circumstances, Stanley Hauerwas and Richard Bondi come closer to holding that the distinction requires certain theological or quasi-theological convictions. See Stanley Hauerwas with Richard Bondi, "Memory, Community, and the Reasons for Living: Reflections on Suicide and Euthanasia," in *Truthfulness and Tragedy* (University of Notre Dame Press, 1977), pp. 101–115.

5. Joseph Heller, *Something Happened* (Ballantine Books, 1975), p. 39. For an analysis of trust, see James F. Childress, "Nonviolent Resistance: Trust and Risk-Taking," *Journal of Religious Ethics,* Fall 1973, pp. 87–112.

6. David Louisell, "Euthanasia and Biothanasia: On Dying and Killing," *Linacre Quarterly,* Vol. 40 (1973), p. 243.

7. See, for example, Jack Cady, "The Burning," *Atlantic Monthly,* August 1965. Much of the current interest in controlling pain in the process of dying centers in the hospice movement.

8. See Robert M. Veatch, *Death, Dying, and the Biological Revolution: Our Last Quest for Responsibility* (Yale University Press, 1976), pp. 97–99, and Ramsey, *Ethics at the Edges of Life,* p. 217.

9. Gerald Kelly, S.J., "The Duty to Preserve Life," *Theological Studies,* December 1951, p. 550. See also the discussions of ordinary and extraordinary means of treatment in Paul Ramsey, *The Patient as Person: Explorations in Medical Ethics* (Yale University Press, 1970), Ch. 3; Ramsey, *Ethics at the Edges of Life,* Ch. 4, where he reduces the morally important meaning of the ordinary/extraordinary distinction "almost without significant remainder to a medical indications policy" (p. 155); and Veatch, *Death, Dying, and the Biological Revolution,* Ch. 3. According to both Ramsey and Veatch, we should abandon the language of ordinary and extraordinary means of prolonging life. Veatch's main reason is that its unclarity makes it unusable as a basis of policy; Ramsey's main reason is that its contemporary use or misuse leads to active, involuntary euthanasia.

10. Another distinction that is sometimes proposed for *how* death is brought about is morally irrelevant. This is the distinction between *withholding* treatment that has not been started (e.g., not resuscitating a patient) and *withdrawing* treatment that has been started (e.g., disconnecting a respirator). However important this distinction may be psychologically, it has no moral significance. Often it is important to begin treatment (e.g., the use of a respirator) in order to gain time for diagnosis and prognosis.

11. Jean Renoir, *The Rules of the Game: A Film,* tr. from the French by John McGrath and Maureen Teitelbaum (Simon & Schuster, 1970).

12. Charles Fried, "Terminating Life Support: Out of the Closet!" *New England Journal of Medicine,* Aug. 12, 1976, p. 390. In that same issue are "Optimum Care for Hopelessly Ill Patients: A Report of the Clinical Care Committee of the Massachusetts General Hospital"; Mitchell T. Rabkin, Gerald Gillerman, and Nancy R. Rice, "Orders Not to Resuscitate"; and Sissela Bok, "Personal Directions for Care at the End of Life," on which Fried comments.

13. Raymond S. Duff, "On Deciding the Use of the Family Commons," in Daniel Bergsma and Ann E. Pulver (eds.), *Developmental Disabilities: Psychologic and Social Implications.* Birth Defects: Original Article Series, Vol. 12, No. 4 (Alan R. Liss, 1976), p. 79. Duff's idea

of the "commons" is drawn from Garrett Hardin, "The Tragedy of the Commons," *Science,* Vol. 162 (1968), pp. 1243–1248. See also Raymond S. Duff and A. G. M. Campbell, "Moral and Ethical Dilemmas in the Special-Care Nursery," *New England Journal of Medicine,* Oct. 25, 1973, pp. 890–894, and "On Deciding the Care of Severely Handicapped or Dying Persons: With Particular Reference to Infants," *Pediatrics,* Vol. 57 (1976), pp. 487–493.

14. For these criteria, see James F. Childress, "Just-War Theories: The Bases, Interrelations, Priorities and Functions of Their Criteria," *Theological Studies,* September 1978, pp. 427–445. For their application to the care of defective newborns, see David H. Smith, "On Letting Some Babies Die," *Hastings Center Studies,* May 1974, pp. 37–46.

15. Both Veatch and Ramsey support some version of living will legislation. Their reasons are very different in part because Veatch stresses liberty and Ramsey stresses equality. Veatch favors legislation authorizing living wills in order to allow individuals to express their preferences and values. Ramsey supports carefully drawn legislation, such as the California statute (with some exceptions), because of his political judgment that it may be the last chance to resist the tide toward a general practice of involuntary euthanasia. This legislation, he suggests, can be helpful if it is "narrowly drawn to encompass only allowing the *dying* to die" (Ramsey, *Ethics at the Edges of Life,* p. 329). See Veatch, *Death, Dying, and the Biological Revolution,* Ch. 5. Contrast Richard A. McCormick and André E. Hellegers, "Legislation and the Living Will," *America,* March 12, 1977, pp. 210–213; they argue that such legislation tends to restrict the rights of both patients and physicians.

16. Richard A. McCormick, S.J., "To Save or Let Die: The Dilemma of Modern Medicine," *Journal of the American Medical Association,* Vol. 229, No. 8 (1974), pp. 172–177, and "The Quality of Life, the Sanctity of Life," *Hastings Center Report,* February 1978.

17. Marc Lappé, "What Counts in Deciding to Withhold Treatment from the Defective Newborn?" *Tufts Medical Alumni Bulletin,* June 1974. For physicians' attitudes, see Diana Crane, "Physicians' Attitudes Toward the Treatment of Critically Ill Patients," in John A. Behnke and Sissela Bok (eds.), *The Dilemmas of Euthanasia* (Doubleday & Co., Anchor Book, 1975), pp. 117–120. For a helpful analysis of "quality of life," see Anthony Shaw, "Defining the Quality of Life," *Hastings Center Report,* October 1977, p. 11.

18. See Joseph Fletcher, *Humanhood: Essays in Biomedical Ethics* (Prometheus Books, 1979), Ch. 1.

19. Ramsey, *Ethics at the Edges of Life,* p. 172.

20. *In the Matter of Earle Spring,* 405 N.E. 2d 115 Mass. 1980. This case is discussed by George J. Annas, "Quality of Life in the Courts: Earle Spring in Fantasyland," *Hastings Center Report,* August 1980, pp. 9–10. See also the articles by Fred Barbash in *The Washington Post,* Jan. 23 and 24, 1980. Annas' "Denying the Rights of the Retarded: The Phillip Becker Case," *Hastings Center Report,* December 1979, pp. 18–20, is also helpful.

21. Ramsey, *Ethics at the Edges of Life,* pp. 157–187. Ramsey fears that Veatch's emphasis on liberty and autonomy would lead to a voluntaristic conception of values and patients' claims and make physicians into automatons.

22. John Updike, *Couples* (Fawcett World Library, 1970), p. 399.

23. The basic structure of this chapter derives from my lecture to the Visiting Committee of the University of Chicago Divinity School. It was subsequently published as "On Ending Life," *Criterion,* Summer 1978, pp. 4–8, and is used by permission. It also incorporates some materials from my "To Kill or Let Die," in Elsie L. Bandman and Bertram Bandman (eds.), *Bioethics and Human Rights: A Reader for Health Professionals* (Little, Brown & Co., 1978), pp. 128–131, and my "Ethical Issues in Death and Dying," *Religious Studies Review,* July 1978, pp. 180–188, a bibliographical essay on books and articles from 1974 to early 1978, with an emphasis on Veatch and Ramsey. Versions of this chapter have been presented in several different settings: Swarthmore College, The College of William and Mary, Augustana College, Texas Medical Center (under the auspices of the Institute of Religion), Lehigh University, Long Island University, Uniformed Services Medical Center, and Hastings Center Workshops. I express my gratitude to these institutions, to their representatives who arranged my visits, and to individuals who offered criticisms and suggestions.

CHAPTER 3
HUMAN SUBJECTS IN RESEARCH

1. For these codes of research ethics, see Beauchamp and Childress, *Principles of Biomedical Ethics,* Appendix II.

2. Henry Beecher, "Ethics and Clinical Research," *New England Journal of Medicine,* Vol. 274 (1966), pp. 1354–1360. See also Henry Beecher, *Research and the Individual: Human Studies* (Little, Brown & Co., 1970).

3. See James Jones, *Bad Blood: The Tuskegee Study of Untreated Syphilis in the Negro Male* (Free Press, 1981).

4. These models are ideal types and thus represent tendencies rather than any particular thinker's ideas. Nevertheless, Joseph Fletcher comes very close to the consequentialist model as I have described it. See Fletcher, "Experiments on Humans," in *Humanhood: Essays in Biomedical Ethics*, pp. 177–189, and, for his general method, *Situation Ethics: The New Morality* (Westminster Press, 1966).

5. See Hans Jonas, "Philosophical Reflections on Experimenting with Human Subjects," *Daedalus*, Spring 1969, and Ramsey, *The Patient as Person*, esp. Ch. 1.

6. See Charles Fried, *Medical Experimentation: Personal Integrity and Social Policy* (American Elsevier Publishing Co., 1974).

7. Ronald Dworkin, *Taking Rights Seriously*, p. xi.

8. This theme pervades Paul Ramsey's writings; see, for example, *War and the Christian Conscience: How Shall Modern War Be Conducted Justly?* (Duke University Press, 1961), Ch. 1.

9. See Stanley Milgram, *Obedience to Authority: An Experimental View* (Harper & Row, 1974).

10. For the controversy, see James J. McCartney, "Encephalitis and Ara-A: An Ethical Case Study," *Hastings Center Report*, December 1978, pp. 5–7, and the response by R. J. Whitley, C. A. Alford, and the NIAID (National Institute of Allergy and Infectious Diseases) Collaborative Antiviral Study Group, *Hastings Center Report*, August 1979, pp. 4, 44–46, accompanied by a response by McCartney (p. 47).

11. Code of Federal Regulations, Title 45, U.S. Code, Part 46, revised as of November 16, 1978.

12. For other discussions of criteria for ethically justified research, see LeRoy Walters, "Some Ethical Issues in Research Involving Human Subjects," *Perspectives in Biology and Medicine*, Winter 1977, pp. 193–211, and Karen Lebacqz, "Controlled Clinical Trials: Some Ethical Issues," *Controlled Clinical Trials*, May 1980, pp. 29–36.

13. Jonas, "Philosophical Reflections on Experimenting with Human Subjects," pp. 224–237.

14. See Bradford H. Gray, *Human Subjects in Medical Experimentation* (Wiley-Interscience, 1975); Amelia L. Schultz and Geraldine P. Pardee, "Are Research Subjects Really Informed?" *Western Journal of Medicine*, Vol. 123 (1975), pp. 76–80; Harmon L. Smith, "Myocardial Infarction—Case Studies of Ethics in the Consent Situation," *Social Science and Medicine*, Vol. 8 (1974), pp. 399–404; and John Fletcher, "Realities of Patient Consent to Medical Research," *Hastings Center Studies*, Vol. 1, No. 1 (1973), pp. 39–49.

15. *Halushka* v. *University of Saskatchewan,* 52 W.W.R. 608 (Sask. C.A. 1965) reprinted in Jay Katz, *Experimentation with Human Beings* (Russell Sage Foundation, 1972), pp. 569–573.

16. John Stuart Mill, *On Liberty* (Penguin Books, 1976), p. 173.

17. Richard A. McCormick, S.J., "Experimental Subjects: Who Should They Be?" *Journal of the American Medical Association,* May 17, 1976, p. 2197. See also McCormick, "Proxy Consent in the Experimental Situation," *Perspectives in Biology and Medicine,* Autumn 1974, pp. 2–20.

18. See Arnold S. Tannenbaum and Robert A. Cooke, "Research in Prisons: A Preliminary Report," in National Commission for the Protection of Human Subjects of Biomedical and Behavioral Research, *Research Involving Prisoners,* DHEW Publication No. (OS) 76–132 (1976), pp. 10–46.

19. Alvin Bronstein's comments, in *Experiments and Research with Humans: Values in Conflict* (Washington, D.C.: National Academy of Sciences, 1975), p. 134.

20. See Carl Cohen, "Medical Experimentation on Prisoners," *Perspectives in Biology and Medicine,* Spring 1978, pp. 357–372. For a legal discussion, see George J. Annas, Leonard H. Glantz, and Barbara F. Katz, *Informed Consent to Human Experimentation: The Subject's Dilemma* (Ballinger Publishing Co., 1977), Ch. 4.

21. Tannenbaum and Cooke, "Research in Prisons," pp. 10–56.

22. See Walter Pincus, "The Federal Register," *The Washington Post,* June 16, 1980, p. A16.

23. National Commission for the Protection of Human Subjects of Biomedical and Behavioral Research, *Research Involving Prisoners, Report and Recommendations,* DHEW Publication No. (OS) 76–131 (1976).

24. See Jonas, "Philosophical Reflections on Experimenting with Human Subjects," pp. 237–243. For the most thorough and helpful examination of clinical trials, see Fried, *Medical Experimentation.*

25. The Danish Obesity Project, "Randomised Trial of Jejunoileal Bypass Versus Medical Treatment in Morbid Obesity," *The Lancet,* Dec. 15, 1979, p. 1255.

26. See Norman Fost, "A Surrogate System for Informed Consent," *Journal of the American Medical Association,* Aug. 18, 1975, pp. 800–803. Unfortunately he sometimes refers to it as "a possible alternative mechanism" to "informed consent." See p. 800.

27. See Fried, *Medical Experimentation,* esp. pp. 160–165.

28. Philippe V. Cardon et al., "Injuries to Research Subjects: A

128 NOTES

Survey of Investigators," *New England Journal of Medicine,* Sept. 16, 1976, pp. 650–654.

29. See Clark Havighurst, "Compensating Persons Injured in Human Experimentation," *Science,* July 10, 1970, pp. 153–157. I do not deal with compensation for participation in research. Such compensation should probably be for time and inconvenience, rather than participation, and it should not constitute an "undue incentive."

30. Bernard R. Adams and Marilyn Shea-Stonum, "Toward a Theory of Control of Medical Experimentation with Human Subjects: The Role of Compensation," *Case Western Reserve Law Review,* Spring 1975, pp. 637ff.

31. Perhaps even research that is not directly sponsored or mandated could be construed as meeting this test, but I will not try to develop that argument now. The argument could take the following direction: "The researching physician stands in a position analogous to an agent for the society. Society desires increases in medical knowledge; it entrusts to the medical profession responsibility for deciding what tests with human subjects should be made, how they should be conducted, and who should be recruited as participants. When a physician decides, pursuant to this trust, to subject a diseased person to unknown risks primarily for society's benefit, and not solely for the patient's own good, society incurs an obligation to compensate for a resulting injury." ("Medical Experiment Insurance," *Columbia Law Review,* May 1970, pp. 977–998.)

32. The term "injury" is ambiguous, for it may refer to harm, disability, or death, on the one hand, or to injustices and wrongs, on the other. While people can be harmed by actions to which they consent, we often hold that no legal or moral wrong has been done to someone who consented to an action. Nevertheless, for various reasons society may refuse to recognize the consent of the victim as a defense to a charge of mayhem or murder. In the context of this chapter, the *volenti* maxim is construed as a denial of a right of recovery for harm, disability, or death—in the absence of negligence—if the research subject has consented to the risks of the experiment. For discussion of the *volenti* maxim, see Joel Feinberg, "Legal Paternalism," *Canadian Journal of Philosophy,* Vol. 1, No. 1 (1971), pp. 105–124.

33. See H. Tristram Engelhardt, Jr., "A Study of the Federal Government's Ethical Obligations to Provide Compensation . . . ," *HEW Secretary's Task Force on the Compensation of Injured Research Subjects,* DHEW Publication No. (OS) 77–004 (1977), Appendix A, pp. 45–63.

34. *HEW Secretary's Task Force on the Compensation of Injured Research*

Subjects, DHEW Publication No. (OS) 77–003 (1977), Report, VI-9.

35. Much of this section on compensation is drawn by permission from my article "Compensating Injured Research Subjects: I. The Moral Argument," *Hastings Center Report,* December 1976, pp. 21–27, which grew out of an oral presentation that I made to the DHEW Secretary's Task Force on the Compensation of Injured Research Subjects, October 16, 1975. LeRoy Walters, who also presented a paper to the Task Force, Charles McCarthy, a member of the Task Force, and Kenneth Casebeer were very helpful in discussions of several points, although they are not, of course, responsible for the use I made of their suggestions. The basic theses of this chapter were originally presented in a Seminar on Biomedical Ethics at the National Institutes of Health (September 1975) and at Connecticut College (February 1976). (For the latter, see my "Ethical Issues in Experimentation with Human Subjects," *Connecticut Medicine,* October 1979, pp. 26–31, from which several paragraphs, especially in the sections on models and criteria, have been drawn.) These theses were further developed in a course on "Issues in Human Experimentation," which I co-taught with Professor Patricia King at the Georgetown University Law School, and in a lecture on "Is All Information Required for Informed Consent?" at the First Annual Meeting of the Society for Clinical Trials (May 1980). I am grateful to participants in all these settings and particularly to Patricia King for illuminating discussions.

CHAPTER 4
ALLOCATING HEALTH CARE RESOURCES

1. Thomas R. Dye, *Understanding Public Policy,* 2d ed. (Prentice-Hall, 1975), p. 1.

2. For an examination of *processes* in "tragic choices," see Guido Calabresi and Philip Bobbitt, *Tragic Choices* (W. W. Norton & Co., 1978), particularly their emphasis on openness and honesty in processes of allocation.

3. Rawls, *A Theory of Justice.* For instance, Ronald M. Green accepts Rawls's theory, with some modifications, and develops its implications for health care policy. ("Health Care and Justice in Contract Theory Perspective," in *Ethics and Health Policy,* Robert M. Veatch and Roy Branson, eds., [Ballinger Publishing Co., 1976], Ch. 7.)

4. Albert R. Jonsen and Lewis H. Butler, "Public Ethics and Policy Making," *Hastings Center Report,* August 1975, pp. 19–31.

5. There is some confusion between the *needs principle* and the

equal-access principle perhaps even in Gene Outka's fine discussion in
"Social Justice and Equal Access to Health Care," *Journal of Religious
Ethics,* Spring 1974, pp. 11–32. As Albert Weale notes, it is possible
to satisfy needs up to an equal level in a society without satisfying
needs as such. For example, providing extra police protection for an
individual who is at grave risk may give him the same level of security
as his fellow citizens, but the need for security by this individual and
the whole community may still not be met. The satisfaction of needs,
including the need for health care, thus must be distinguished from
the provision of equal access to what society provides to meet those
needs. See Albert Weale, *Equality and Social Policy* (London: Rout-
ledge & Kegan Paul, 1978). I discuss Outka's position in relation to
this distinction in "A Right to Health Care?" *Journal of Medicine and
Philosophy,* June 1979, where I also examine other issues of relevance
to priorities in the allocation of resources for and within health care.

   6. Rick J. Carlson, "Alternative Legislative Strategies for Licensure:
Licensure and Health." Paper presented at the Conference on Quality
Assurance in Hospitals, Boston University, Program on Public Policy
for Quality Health Care, Nov. 21–22, 1975. Quoted by Walter J.
McNerney, "The Quandary of Quality Assessment," *New England
Journal of Medicine,* Dec. 30, 1976, p. 1507. See also Rick J. Carlson,
The End of Medicine (John Wiley & Sons, 1975).

   7. See Ivan Illich, *Medical Nemesis: The Expropriation of Health* (London: Calder and Boyars, 1975).

   8. Paul Starr, "The Politics of Therapeutic Nihilism," *Hastings
Center Report,* October 1976, pp. 24–30.

   9. For a similar list of priority questions, see Outka, "Social Justice
and Equal Access to Health Care," p. 29, fn. 5. For the first two
questions it is often difficult to determine whether and where in the
public policy process there is a direct conflict between health care and
other social goods or between prevention and rescue. The process is
very complicated, and my discussion should not be taken to imply that
these choices are present in a clear and manageable form. Nevertheless, some policies reflect these choices, and an attempt to offer a
moral illumination of some of the issues may also suggest that the
process needs altering so that they can be confronted clearly and
directly.

   10. For the distinction between "first-order" and "second-order"
determinations, see Calabresi and Bobbitt, *Tragic Choices.*

   11. Antony Flew, "Ends and Means," in Paul Edwards (ed.), *The
Encyclopedia of Philosophy* (Macmillan Co., 1967), Vol. 2, p. 510.

   12. Ramsey, *The Patient as Person,* pp. 240, 268. By contrast,
Ronald Green argues that the question of how much the society

should spend on health should be handled in terms of general moral principles rather than left to the political process. Within contract theory, he contends, "members of the original position as the architects of the basic social system want to set some upper and lower limits on the availability of health services." Green's argument depends on a modification of Rawls's theory of primary goods to include health under the "social primary goods" rather than under the "natural primary goods" whose distribution is only indirectly affected by the social structure. See "Health Care and Justice in Contract Theory Perspective," in Veatch and Branson (eds.), *Ethics and Health Policy.*

13. Charles Fried, "Equality and Rights in Medical Care," *Implications of Guaranteeing Medical Care* in Joseph G. Perpich (ed.), (Washington, D.C.: National Academy of Sciences, Institute of Medicine, 1976), pp. 3–14.

14. Lewis Thomas, "Rx for Illich," *The New York Review of Books,* Sept. 16, 1976, pp. 3–4, and *The Lives of a Cell: Notes of a Biology Watcher* (Viking Press, 1974), pp. 31–36.

15. U.S. Department of Health, Education, and Welfare. Public Health Service, *Forward Plan for Health:* FY 1977–81 (DHEW Publication No. OS-76-50024), p. 15. Cf. Marc LaLonde, *A New Perspective on the Health of Canadians: A Working Document* (Ottawa, Canada: The Government of Canada, 1974).

16. These categories and figures are presented in Michael S. Koleda et al., *The Federal Health Dollar: 1969–1976* (Washington, D.C.: National Planning Association, Center for Health Policy Studies, 1977).

17. Thomas Schelling, "The Life You Save May Be Your Own," Samuel B. Chase, Jr. (ed.), in *Problems in Public Expenditure Analysis* (Washington, D.C.: The Brookings Institution, 1966), pp. 127–166.

18. Charles Fried, *An Anatomy of Values: Problems of Personal and Social Choice* (Harvard University Press, 1970), pp. 224f. Fried's argument is important for much of this section of this chapter.

19. See Max Weber, *Max Weber on Law in Economy and Society,* ed. and anno. by Max Rheinstein and tr. by Edward Shils and Max Rheinstein (Simon & Schuster, 1967), p. 1. The translators use the term "purpose-rational" for *zweckrational.*

20. Richard Zeckhauser, "Procedures for Valuing Lives," *Public Policy,* Fall 1975, pp. 447–448. Contrast Richard A. Rettig, "Valuing Lives: The Policy Debate on Patient Care Financing for Victims of End-Stage Renal Disease," *The Rand Paper Series* (Santa Monica, Calif.: The Rand Corporation, 1976).

21. Fried, *An Anatomy of Values,* p. 217.

22. Lawrence C. Becker, "The Neglect of Virtue," *Ethics,* January 1975, pp. 110–122. See also Lewis H. LaRue, "A Comment on Fried,

Summers, and the Value of Life," *Cornell Law Review*, Vol. 57, (1972), pp. 621–631, and Benjamin Freedman, "The Case for Medical Care, Inefficient or Not," *Hastings Center Report*, April 1977, pp. 31–39.

23. For a fuller discussion of compensatory justice, see Ch. 3 and Childress, "Compensating Injured Research Subjects: I. The Moral Argument," pp. 21–27. Cf. also Fried, *An Anatomy of Values*, p. 220.

24. See Milton C. Weinstein and William B. Stason, "Allocating Resources: The Case of Hypertension." *Hastings Center Report*, October 1977, pp. 24–29; "Allocation of Resources to Manage Hypertension," *New England Journal of Medicine*, Vol. 296 (1977), pp. 732–739; and *Hypertension: A Policy Perspective* (Harvard University Press, 1976). Recent data indicate that "the stroke death rate, when adjusted for age changes in the population, has declined 36.1 percent since 1962, with more than two-thirds of that drop occurring since 1972, the year a major, continuing national campaign was begun to identify and treat those suffering from high blood pressure" (B. D. Colen, "Deaths Caused by Strokes Fall Sharply in U.S.," *The Washington Post*, Feb. 23, 1979, pp. A1, A9).

25. Outka, "Social Justice and Equal Access to Health Care," p. 24.

26. Conrad Taeuber, "If Nobody Died of Cancer . . ." *The Kennedy Institute Quarterly Report*, Summer 1976, pp. 6–9.

27. Franz J. Ingelfinger, "Haves and Have-Nots in the World of Disease," *New England Journal of Medicine*, Dec. 7, 1972, pp. 1198–1199.

28. Jay Katz and Alexander Morgan Capron, *Catastrophic Diseases: Who Decides What?* (Russell Sage Foundation, 1975), p. 178.

29. Leon Kass, "Regarding the End of Medicine and the Pursuit of Health," *The Public Interest*, Summer 1975, p. 39.

30. See Nedra B. Belloc and Lester Breslow, "Relationship of Physical Status and Health Practices," *Preventive Medicine*, Vol. 1 (1972), pp. 409–421, and Nedra B. Belloc, "Relationship of Health Practices and Mortality," *Preventive Medicine*, Vol. 2 (1973), pp. 67–81.

31. Victor R. Fuchs, *Who Shall Live? Health, Economics, and Social Choice* (Basic Books, 1974), p. 53 (italics added).

32. Fried, *An Anatomy of Values*, Pt. III, Chs. 10–12.

33. These quotations from Hecaton's "Moral Duties" appear in Cicero, *De Officiis*, tr. by Walter Miller (Harvard University Press, 1947), p. 365.

34. Ambrose, *Duties of the Clergy*, III. 4, Nicene and Post-Nicene Fathers of the Christian Church, Second Series, Vol. 10 (New York: The Christian Literature Company, 1896), p. 71. See also Lactantius'

discussion of the so-called "board of Carneades" in *The Divine Institutes,* The Fathers of the Church, A New Translation, Vol. 49 (Catholic University of America Press, 1964), V 17.

35. See Saul Lieberman, "How Much Greek in Jewish Palestine?" in Alexander Altmann (ed.), *Biblical and Other Studies* (Harvard University Press, 1963), pp. 124–127. For further discussions, see Chaim W. Reines, "The Self and the Other in Rabbinic Ethics," and Louis Jacobs, "Greater Love Hath No Man . . . The Jewish Point of View of Self-Sacrifice," in Menachem Marc Kellner (ed.), *Contemporary Jewish Ethics* (Sanhedrin Press Book, Hebrew Publishing Co., 1978), and Jakob J. Petuchowski, "The Limits of Self-Sacrifice," in Marvin Fox, (ed.), *Modern Jewish Ethics* (Ohio State University Press, 1975).

36. See, for example, *United States* v. *Holmes* 26 Fed. Cas 360 (No. 15383) (C.C.E.D. Pa. 1842) and *Regina* v. *Dudley,* 14 Q.B.D. 273 (1884). The former involved jettison, while the latter involved cannibalism. See also Lon Fuller's fictional case, "The Case of the Speluncean Explorers," *Harvard Law Review,* Vol. 62 (1949), pp. 616–645.

37. Ramsey, *The Patient as Person,* p. 254. The lifeboat has been used as a metaphor by Garrett Hardin, who discusses world hunger in terms of "lifeboat ethics." See, for example, his "Living on a Lifeboat," *Bioscience,* October 1974, pp. 561–568.

38. Harry S. Abram, Gordon L. Moore, and Frederic B. Westervelt, "Suicidal Behavior in Chronic Dialysis Patients," *American Journal of Psychiatry,* Vol. 127 (1971), pp. 1199–1204.

39. "Scarce Medical Resources," *Columbia Law Review,* April 1969, pp. 654, 656.

40. Nicholas Rescher, "The Allocation of Exotic Medical Lifesaving Therapy," *Ethics,* April 1969, p. 178.

41. See Fried, *Medical Experimentation.*

42. Howard Hiatt, "Protecting the Medical Commons: Who Is Responsible?" *New England Journal of Medicine,* July 31, 1975, pp. 235–241.

43. For a development of the perspective of this paragraph, see Charles Fried, "Rights and Health Care—Beyond Equity and Efficiency," *New England Journal of Medicine,* July 31, 1975, pp. 241–245. For a fuller discussion of the social responsibility of physicians, see Albert R. Jonsen and Andrew L. Jameton, "Social and Political Responsibilities of Physicians," and James F. Childress, "Citizen and Physician: Harmonious or Conflicting Responsibilities?" *Journal of Medicine and Philosophy,* December 1977.

44. Joseph Fletcher, *The Greatest Good of the Greatest Number: A New Frontier in the Morality of Medical Care,* Sanger Lecture, No. 7 (Rich-

mond, Va.: Medical College of Virginia, Virginia Commonwealth University, n.d.).

45. Marc D. Basson, "Choosing Among Candidates for Scarce Medical Resources," *Journal of Medicine and Philosophy*, September 1979, p. 331.

46. Leo Shatin, "Medical Care and the Social Worth of a Man," *American Journal of Orthopsychiatry*, Vol. 36 (1966), pp. 96–101. I should note that I have stated "utilitarian selection" in "act-utilitarian" terms. Part of my argument for the use of impersonal mechanisms hinges on "rule-utilitarian" considerations (e.g., the consequences of adopting such a rule).

47. Ramsey, *The Patient as Person*, p. 259. An argument for a lottery, or some form of chance, does not presuppose convictions about divine activity. Although lots were used in the Old Testament (e.g., to determine why the ship carrying Jonah was sinking) and in the New Testament (e.g., to fill Judas' position among the disciples), it may have a secular rationale too: where God is silent, it may make sense to cast lots. Within the third approach, a lottery is only one way to determine who will receive a scarce resource; queuing and randomization are others. Which is preferable will depend on several factors, including feasibility. For example, queuing may be more feasible for some forms of critical care because people's needs develop at different times. But people may seek treatment at different times because of injustice in the system; for example, some patients may not get in line early because of lack of information or even overt discrimination.

48. For other reasons, see James F. Childress, "Who Shall Live When Not All Can Live?" *Soundings*, Winter 1970, pp. 339–355 (reprinted in various books). For other defenses of the use of chance, see Jay Katz and Alexander Morgan Capron, *Catastrophic Diseases: Who Decides What?*, esp. pp. 184–196. See also the recommendation of the Artificial Heart Assessment Panel of the National Heart and Lung Institute: "In the event artificial heart resources are in scarce supply, decisions as to the selection of candidates for implantation of the artificial heart should be made by physicians and medical institutions on the basis of medical criteria. If the pool of patients with equal medical needs exceeds supply, procedures should be devised for some form of random selection. Social worth criteria should not be used, and every effort should be exerted to minimize the possibility that social worth may implicitly be taken into account." (*The Totally Implantable Artificial Heart*, June 1973, DHEW Publication No. [NIH] 74–191, p. 198.) For an imaginative presentation of the issues, see George J. Annas, "Allocation of Artificial Hearts in the Year 2002:

Minerva v. *National Health Agency,*" *American Journal of Law and Medicine,* Vol. 3, No. 1 (1977), pp. 59–76.

49. Rescher, "The Allocation of Exotic Medical Life-saving Therapy," p. 183.

50. Ramsey, *The Patient as Person,* pp. 257–258.

51. *Ibid.* For a discussion of triage, see Thomas J. O'Donnell, S.J., "The Morality of Triage," *The Georgetown Medical Bulletin,* August 1960, pp. 68–71.

52. "Scarce Medical Resources," p. 664.

53. The first three sections of this chapter are reprinted, with modifications, by permission from *Soundings,* Fall 1979, pp. 256–274. The fourth section on microallocation incorporates by permission several paragraphs from my article "Rationing of Medical Treatment," in Warren T. Reich (ed.), *Encyclopedia of Bioethics,* Vol. 4 (Free Press, 1978), pp. 1414–1419. The formulation and development of the ideas and arguments in this chapter benefited greatly from discussions at many colleges, universities, medical schools, and other institutions. Among the most fruitful discussions were those at the University of Tennessee (Knoxville), the Center for Disease Control, the National Institutes of Health, the School of Public Health of the University of North Carolina at Chapel Hill, the Albert Einstein College of Medicine of Yeshiva University, the Institute of Religion at the Texas Medical Center, Princeton Theological Seminary, and Indiana University, which subsequently reproduced and circulated one version of this chapter. I am grateful to the persons at these and other institutions who sponsored my lectures and who contributed incisive criticisms and suggestions.

CHAPTER 5
THE ART OF TECHNOLOGY ASSESSMENT

1. See Harvey Cox, *The Secular City* (Macmillan Co. 1965); Daniel Bell, *The End of Ideology* (Free Press of Glencoe, 1960), especially "An Epilogue: The End of Ideology in the West"; and Peter Laslett (ed.), *Philosophy, Politics and Society,* First Series (Oxford: Basil Blackwell, Publisher, 1957), "Introduction."

2. Arthur Schlesinger, Jr., *A Thousand Days* (Houghton Mifflin Co., 1965), p. 644. See also William Lee Miller, *Of Thee, Nevertheless, I Sing* (Harcourt Brace Jovanovich, 1975), pp. 78–95. These themes were

prominent in President Kennedy's commencement speech at Yale University in 1962.

3. Jacques Ellul, *The Technological Society,* tr. from the French by John Wilkinson (Vintage Books, 1964).

4. Daniel J. Boorstin, *The Republic of Technology: Reflections on Our Future Community* (Harper & Row, 1978).

5. Stanley Joel Reiser, *Medicine and the Reign of Technology* (Cambridge University Press, 1978).

6. This definition is a modification of the definition offered in *Assessing Biomedical Technologies: An Inquiry Into the Nature of the Process,* by the Committee on the Life Sciences and Social Policy, National Research Council (Washington, D.C.: National Academy of Sciences, 1975), p. 1.

7. The term "control" is anathema to many critics of contemporary society and technology, perhaps especially in religious contexts; some critics have retreated into the private sphere because technology appears to be out of control or because the issues are thought to be cultural rather than political. For a valuable discussion of "autonomous technology," see Langdon Winner, *Autonomous Technology: Technics-out-of-Control as a Theme in Political Thought* (MIT Press, 1977).

8. Joseph F. Coates, "The Identification and Selection of Candidates and Priorities for Technology Assessment," *Technology Assessment,* Vol. 2, No. 2 (1974), p. 78. For an overview of technology assessment, see LeRoy Walters, "Technology Assessment," in Reich (ed.), *Encyclopedia of Bioethics,* Vol. 4, pp. 1650–1654.

9. See James M. Gustafson, *The Contributions of Theology to Medical Ethics,* The 1975 Pere Marquette Theology Lecture (Marquette University Press, 1975). In a critique of most, if not all, theological approaches to technology and the life sciences, Gustafson castigates casuists and moralists for their myopia and prophetic theologians for their inability to deal with specifics. See James M. Gustafson, "Theology Confronts Technology and the Life Sciences," *Commonweal,* June 16, 1978, pp. 386–392.

10. Weber drew the phrase "disenchantment of the world" *(Entzauberung der Welt)* from Friedrich Schiller. See Max Weber, *The Protestant Ethic and the Spirit of Capitalism,* tr. by Talcott Parsons (Charles Scribner's Sons, 1958), esp. pp. 105 and 221–222, fn. 19, and H. H. Gerth and C. Wright Mills (eds.), *From Max Weber: Essays in Sociology* (Oxford University Press, 1958), p. 51.

11. Lynn White, Jr., "The Historical Roots of Our Ecologic Crisis," *Science,* March 10, 1967.

12. Gerhard Liedke, "Solidarity in Conflict," in *Faith and Science in an Unjust World: Report of the World Council of Churches' Conference on*

Faith, Science and the Future, Vol. 1, Plenary Presentations, ed. by Roger Shinn (Fortress Press, 1980), pp. 73–80. In contrast, Charles Birch's presentation in the same volume stresses oneness and harmony and calls for a process theology ("Nature, Humanity and God in Ecological Perspective," pp. 62–73).

13. For some of these principles, see Beauchamp and Childress, *Principles of Biomedical Ethics.*

14. Calabresi and Bobbitt, *Tragic Choices.*

15. See James F. Childress, "Reflections on Socialist Ethics," and H. Tristram Engelhardt, Jr., "Bioethical Issues in Contemporary China," *The Kennedy Institute Quarterly Report,* Fall 1979, pp. 11–14 and 4–6.

16. Mill, "Bentham," in Warnock (ed.), *Utilitarianism, On Liberty, Essay on Bentham,* pp. 92 and 105.

17. Warren Weaver, "Statistical Morality," *Christianity and Crisis,* Jan. 23, 1961, pp. 210–215. In the last chapter, I introduced Thomas Schelling's idea of "statistical lives." For a fuller analysis of risk, see James F. Childress, "Risk," in Reich (ed.), *Encyclopedia of Bioethics,* Vol. 4, pp. 1516–1522.

18. For a discussion, see George I. Mavrodes, "The Morality of Chances: Weighing the Cost of Auto Safety," *The Reformed Journal,* March 1980, pp. 12–15.

19. See Steven E. Rhoads (ed.), *Valuing Life: Public Policy Dilemmas* (Westview Press, 1980), especially his chapter "How Much Should We Spend to Save a Life?" pp. 285–311. His formulations have shaped this paragraph.

20. These are Charles Fried's terms as introduced in the previous chapter.

21. Rhoads, "How Much Should We Spend to Save a Life?" pp. 305–306.

22. Harold P. Green, "The Risk-Benefit Calculus in Safety Determinations," *George Washington Law Review,* Vol. 43 (1975), p. 799.

23. James M. Gustafson, "Basic Ethical Issues in the Biomedical Fields," *Soundings,* Summer 1970, p. 153.

24. National Academy of Sciences, Panel on Technology Assessment, *Technology: Processes of Assessment and Choice.* Report to the Committee on Science and Astronautics, U.S. House of Representatives, July 1969 (Washington, D.C.: Government Printing Office, 1969), pp. 33–39.

25. For a defense of "intermediate technologies," see E. F. Schumacher, *Small Is Beautiful* (Harper & Row, 1973); for a defense of "alternative technology," see David Dickson, *The Politics of Alternative Technology* (Universe Books, 1975). For a critique of these move-

ments, see Witold Rybczynski, *Paper Heroes: A Review of Appropriate Technology* (Doubleday & Co., 1980).

26. National Academy of Sciences, *Technology: Processes of Assessment and Choice,* p. 32.

27. Advisory Committee on the Biological Effects of Ionizing Radiations, National Research Council, *Considerations of Health Benefit-Cost Analysis for Activities Involving Ionizing Radiation Exposure and Alternatives* (Washington, D.C.: National Academy of Sciences, 1977), p. 150.

28. Weber, *Max Weber on Law in Economy and Society,* p. 1. It should also be obvious from my argument that I believe that it is both possible and desirable to have rational deliberation about the ends that are chosen. They are not merely arbitrary. Yet, as I suggested in Chapter 4, the selection of some ends is mainly political or even aesthetic.

29. Laurence Tribe, "Technology Assessment and the Fourth Discontinuity: The Limits of Instrumental Rationality," *Southern California Law Review,* June 1973, pp. 657, 634–635. See also Laurence Tribe, "Policy Science: Analysis or Ideology," *Philosophy and Public Affairs,* Fall 1972, pp. 66–110. Tribe's discussion has been important for this chapter, especially for this paragraph and the previous one. For another critique of the assumptions of much technology assessment, see Carroll Pursell, "Belling the Cat, Critique of Technology Assessment," *Lex et Scientia,* Oct.–Dec. 1974, pp. 130–145.

30. See James D. Carroll, "Participatory Technology," *Science,* Vol. 171 (1971), pp. 647–653.

31. Philip Potter, "Science and Technology: Why Are the Churches Concerned?" in *Faith and Science in an Unjust World,* Vol. 1, Plenary Presentations, pp. 26–27. For the reports and recommendations, see *Faith and Science in an Unjust World,* Vol. 2, ed. by Paul Abrecht (Fortress Press, 1980). For a critical analysis of the conference, see Alan Geyer, "The EST Complex at MIT: The Ecumenical-Scientific-Technological Complex," *Ecumenical Review,* October 1979, pp. 372–380, and other essays in that issue (e.g., those by Ian Barbour and Ole Jensen).

32. Harold P. Green, "Cost-Risk-Benefit Assessment and the Law: Introduction and Perspective," *George Washington Law Review,* August 1977, p. 908.

33. For the principle of equal concern and respect, see Ronald Dworkin, *Taking Rights Seriously.*

34. Hans Jonas, "Technology and Responsibility: Reflections on the New Tasks of Ethics," *Philosophical Essays: From Ancient Creed to Technological Man* (Prentice-Hall, 1974), pp. 18–19.

35. Langdon Winner, "On Criticizing Technology," in Albert H. Teich (ed.), *Technology and Man's Future,* 2d ed. (St. Martin's Press, 1977).

36. *Ibid.*

37. Lynn White, Jr., "Technology Assessment from the Stance of a Medieval Historian," *Medieval Religion and Technology: Collected Essays* (University of California Press, 1978), pp. 261–276.

38. This chapter originated in a lecture for a Conference on the Technological Society and the Individual sponsored by the Program on Social and Political Thought at the University of Virginia in 1978. It was subsequently delivered in modified form at Whitworth College (1979), at a symposium on Religious Belief in the Age of Science and Technology sponsored by the Religion Club of the University of Virginia (1980), at Earlham School of Religion as one of the 1980 Willson Lectures, and at Miami University (Ohio) as one of the 1980 Wickenden Lectures. It has been strengthened by various comments and suggestions I received in these settings. I am particularly grateful to Dante Germino who, alas, will not be satisfied that I have answered his criticisms.

INDEX